PUBLIC HEALTH AT THE CROSSROADS

PUBLIC HEALTH
AT THE CROSSROADS

Achievements and prospects

ROBERT BEAGLEHOLE
and
RUTH BONITA

Faculty of Medicine and Health Science
University of Auckland
Auckland
New Zealand

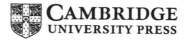
CAMBRIDGE
UNIVERSITY PRESS

PUBLISHED BY THE PRESS SYNDICATE OF THE UNIVERSITY OF CAMBRIDGE
The Pitt Building, Trumpington Street, Cambridge, United Kingdom

CAMBRIDGE UNIVERSITY PRESS
The Edinburgh Building, Cambridge CB2 2RU, UK http://www.cup.cam.ac.uk
40 West 20th Street, New York, NY 10011–4211, USA http://www.cup.org
10 Stamford Road, Oakleigh, Melbourne 3166, Australia

First published 1997
Reprinted 1999

Printed in the United Kingdom at the University Press, Cambridge

Typeface Monotype Times 10/13pt. *System* QuarkXPress® [SE]

A catalogue record for this book is available from the British Library

Library of Congress Cataloguing in Publication data

Beaglehole, R.
    Public health at the crossroads : achievements and prospects /
    Robert Beaglehole and Ruth Bonita.
        p. cm.
    Includes bibliographical references and index.
    ISBN 0 521 58373 X (hardback).   ISBN 0 521 58665 8 (paperback)
    1. World health.   I. Bonita, R.   II. Title.
    [DNLM: 1. World Health.   2. Public Health.   3. Epidemiology.
    4. Health Policy.   WA 530.1 B365p   1997]
    RA441.B43   1997
    362.1   DC21
    DNLM/DLC   96–46126   CIP
    for Library of Congress

ISBN 0 521 58373 X hardback
ISBN 0 521 58665 8 paperback

Contents

Prepublication reviews of Public Health at the Crossroads: Achievements and prospects

Public health really is at a crossroads. Drs Robert Beaglehole and Ruth Bonita trace the origins of the field (the tortuous route we have travelled), the many contemporary challenges (that health really is a global issue) and some future promising directions (how a broader approach to public health grounded in an appropriate epidemiology can inform future social policy). The book is refreshing, truly multidisciplinary, based on relevant data and international in its application. Although given separate attention, the authors highlight the striking structural similarities in the public health problems of the poor and the wealthy countries. *Public Health at the Crossroads* is essential reading for those who wish to look beyond traditional public health and the mechanics of everyday epidemiology to new possibilities and more appropriate strategies and methods.

John B. McKinlay, PhD
Sonja M. McKinlay, PhD
New England Research Institutes
Watertown, MA, USA

This sweeping, panoramic view of the state of health in the world provides a marvellous perspective on the problems of health and disease old and new, among poor and rich nations alike. Again and again the authors zoom in for close-up examinations of the causes of infant and child deaths, the yawning gaps between poor and rich, the historical background and evolutionary development of modern public health movements, capsule summaries of health and the services that provide it, in nations around the world, and much more. Beginning students of public health and epidemiology, those who are midway in their training, and established scholars in the field will learn much from this up-to-the-minute, user-friendly discourse. I recommend it without reservation.

John Last, MD
Emeritus Professor of Epidemiology and
Community Medicine, University of Ottawa, Canada

After a century 'on the road', public health faces important choices. This book examines, in broad social context, the historical journey of public health and its prospects for revitalisation as we enter a new century. Epidemiologists and public health practitioners face a widening challenge: population health problems that range from local to global levels; entrenched social-economic disparities as sources of poor health; and the emerging hazards of a rapidly changing, interdependent world. The book has a fine sense of public health as both a scientific and a social enterprise.

A.J. McMichael
Professor of Epidemiology
London School of Hygiene and Tropical Medicine, UK

Preface

This book assesses the achievements and the current state of epidemiology and public health with a focus on the last 50 years. As we enter the new millennium, the main challenges facing epidemiology and public health are identified and strategies for the future discussed. The main audience for this book is students of epidemiology and public health who will, after all, shape the future of these disciplines.

Public health is the collective action taken by society to protect and promote the health of entire populations; in contrast, clinical medicine deals only with the problems of individuals. Public health is broad and inclusive, although it is often considered from only a narrow medical perspective. Epidemiology, with its focus on the causes of disease at the population level and the methods for their control, is the most important science contributing to public health. Many other disciplines also contribute, for example biostatistics, medical sociology, health economics, and various qualitative approaches. Epidemiology is central to public health because of its population focus and quantitative methods.

Epidemiology and public health are again at a crossroad. The choice is between a narrow focus on health service issues or a refocus on the major causes of population health. The main argument of this book is that both epidemiology and public health are failing to fulfil their potential to improve the public's health. The problem lies both with the public health professions which have narrowed their concerns and because there is a dysjunction between the ideas of public health and the way society organises itself in relation to health.

Despite promising beginnings with Snow and his work on cholera in the middle of the last century, and pathbreaking work a century later on the tobacco-caused lung cancer epidemic, epidemiology is still peripheral to the health endeavour. Internationally, public health has been marginalised as collective responsibility for social welfare in general is replaced by a growing emphasis on market forces and individualism. At the national level, the ongoing debates about health care reforms have been narrowly focused on medical care services and have not embraced the need for a re-emphasis on public health services. Given the endless threats to public health, the prospects for epidemiology and public health will improve only if population health becomes a central concern of the policy making process.

As the purpose of public health is to improve health, this book, which has three main sections, begins with an overview of major health trends and a summary of the current state of the world's health. It also discusses recent estimates of the global burden of disease and identifies the major remaining health problems. This is followed by a discussion of the causes of modern epidemics. The framework for Part I is the health transition and the forces which propel it. Part II describes the development of epidemiology and considers epidemiology's contribution to the improvement in health status. Criticisms of epidemiology are discussed and the major challenges facing epidemiology outlined.

Part III describes the global state of the organisation and delivery of public health services. Case studies of several wealthy countries are used to illustrate different approaches to the organisation of public health activities. In most countries public health has been marginalised and the emphasis is on medical care services. These services know no limit and, with the ageing of the world's population, could easily claim even the small proportion of health budgets spent on public health services. The impact of recent reviews of public health in the United Kingdom, United States of America, Sweden and New Zealand is described. The situation in Japan is outlined because of the major recent health improvements in Japan. In a few poor countries, public health has at various times assumed a more central role in public policy. Two such countries, China and Cuba, have made impressive gains in health status over the last few decades. The third poor country to be considered is India, and here the focus is on the state of Kerala which, despite enduring and widespread poverty, has achieved a remarkably high standard of health.

The book concludes by drawing together the achievements, the present dilemmas and the future prospects for public health; alternative pathways for epidemiology and public health are outlined. Recent worldwide political, economic and environmental changes present the most important challenges to public health in the twenty first century; public health practitioners must adopt a truly global perspective. For epidemiology and public health to move centre stage, it will be necessary to recognise and confront these challenges. A major shift in emphasis is required if public health is to develop with a focus on environmental sustainability, equity and community. This process will be easier if public health practitioners rediscover the reforming values of their nineteenth century predecessors and reconnect with the aspirations and energy of the people and communities they serve. In the short term the initiative must come from public health practitioners. A tremendous responsibility falls on all of us. We need to rediscover our passion for public health so that public health moves forward and fulfils its potential to improve the health of populations globally.

Robert Beaglehole
Ruth Bonita

Acknowledgements

This book had its origins while we were on sabbatical leave from the University of Auckland, New Zealand. We are grateful for this support.

The book has benefited from invaluable feedback from many friends and colleagues to whom we are indebted: in particular Toni Ashton, Peter Davis, Anna Howe, Rod Jackson, Tord Kjellström, Tony McMichael, Alan Norrish, Neil Pearce, George Salmond, David Skegg, Alistair Woodward and Alan Wylie.

Country profiles benefited from input from Kjell Asplund, Warwick Armstrong, Don Bandaranayake, Gilliam Durham, Bobbie Jacobson, Walter Holland, John Powles, Roger Rosenblatt, Hirotsugu Ueshima and Hiroshi Yanagawa.

Sections were written while hosted by Kjell Asplund (Umeå, Sweden), Tord Kjellström (WIIO, Geneva), Alan Lopez (Gryon, Switzerland), Ivan Gyarfas (WHO, Geneva) and Adrienne Taylor (Möens, France).

The mechanics of assembling the material and preparing the manuscript could not have taken place without considerable effort from Joanna Broad, Dale Cormack-Pearson, Raewynne Menzies, Wendy Smidt and Rachael Taylor.

Finally, the preparation of such a manuscript inevitably impacts on family life. We therefore would like to acknowledge the support of our children, Rob Beaglehole and Anna Beaglehole.

Part I
Global health

The first part of this book

- considers the health transition and the forces that propel it (Chapter 1);
- outlines the current state of global health (Chapter 2); and
- describes the major causes of premature death and disease (Chapter 3).

1

Health, disease and the health transition

1.1 Introduction

This Chapter sets the scene by introducing definitions central to an understanding of health and disease, and describes the populations and country
groupings that will be used in our comparisons. It also introduces the health
transition which provides a framework for explaining and describing major
trends in health and disease.

1.2 Health status or disease status?

Health has a wide variety of meanings ranging from an ideal state to the
absence of a medically defined and certified disease. Health as an ideal state
has been encapsulated in the original and inspiratory World Health
Organization (WHO) definition: 'health is a state of complete mental, physical and social well-being and not merely the absence of disease or infirm-
ity'[1]. The definition reflects the optimism at the end of the Second World
War. Unfortunately, health, in this vision, is largely unattainable. While
individuals may occasionally be in this state, populations as a whole will
never be free of premature death, disease or disability because of their close
interaction with a changing environment. The adaptive fit between human
biology and the human-made environment is inevitably imperfect[2].

In the 1980s WHO promoted a more realistic definition of health which
emphasises the ability to function 'normally' in one's own society. 'Health'
here is a means to an end but again requires the absence of disability, disease
or handicap, despite the fact that many people consider themselves to be in
'good health' even in the presence of a disabling disease. By contrast, and
in the opinion of many modern 'health reformers', health is a commodity
which can be 'bought' in discrete packages.

A simple subjective categorisation by individuals into one of three current states of health, for example 'good; fair; poor', has been shown to predict future health outcomes with a surprising degree of accuracy; expectations for health clearly differ between young and old people, and by gender[3]. With further research, this type of subjective information may provide additional dimensions to death statistics. It is not yet useful either for international comparisons or for assessing trends over time. Similarly, measures of health which emphasise 'lived experiences' have had little impact on either epidemiology or public health and are difficult to develop in a standardised manner for comparisons across time or culture[4].

Of more use, both theoretically and practically, is a definition which states that health is created by removing obstacles and by providing the basic means by which individual goals can be achieved[5]. The foundations of health are common to all and include basic requirements such as adequate food, safe water, shelter, safety and hope. In addition, information, education and a sense of community are essential if people are to develop their potential. These foundations have a more profound long-term effect on health status than the activities of the health system[6]. The chosen definition of health has important implications for health policy. It determines whether the emphasis is on a multi-sectoral approach to improving health or whether the focus is on selected diseases and technological solutions[7].

The main source of 'health' data remains death statistics. Epidemiologists are often criticised for concentrating on this narrow aspect of health. Death statistics, however, provide an important starting point because of the gross disparities they reveal and for historical purposes there is no alternative. In addition, death has a deep significance in all societies.

The most useful source of death information is the data supplied to the WHO by member countries. These data depend upon two essential components: an estimate of the population at risk and the identification of deaths. Only a minority of countries conduct regular censuses to determine the age distribution of their populations. Even in wealthy countries such as the United States of America, population counts are not always accurate, especially for minority groups [8].

Counting deaths is even more difficult. Only about 60 of the 187 member states are in a position to provide national death statistics to the WHO[9]. In the absence of national death registration systems for two-third's of the world's population, estimates are used to assess the burden of death[10,11]. A great failure of epidemiology and public health is that insufficient attention has been given to ensuring that adequate vital health data are collected.

As very few countries can provide useful data on deaths going back more than a few decades, trends over time must be interpreted with great caution.

Even the available data are limited by the lack of attention to quality. The problems with death data include:

- changes in diagnostic and death certification fashions;
- periodic revisions of the WHO disease classification system;
- the contribution of multiple causes to death; and
- the generally low and declining use of post-mortems.

Fortunately, many of the known limitations of mortality data tend to cancel out each other and, from a population perspective, the available data are extremely useful in studying overall trends, even if flawed at the individual level. The great attraction of death as a key indicator of health status is that it can be measured more easily than morbidity (sickness). It is often assumed that morbidity changes in parallel with mortality, although this is by no means always true, especially in older people.

Death data are used for a number of purposes. They

- allow comparisons among and within countries;
- demonstrate trends in longevity or life expectancy;
- show trends in death rates for different age groups; and
- provide information about the leading causes of death.

Even a cursory inspection of the available mortality data reveals a tremendous burden of premature death in all countries, especially in poor countries.

1.3 Categorising countries

A striking feature of the global health picture is the great diversity between and, to a lesser extent, within countries. Various classifications are used to group the more than 200 countries in the world, but no system is satisfactory. The World Bank categorises countries according to their gross national product and by eight demographic regions[11]. The regional categories are further simplified into two groups, the former socialist economies of Europe and the established market economies where relatively uniform age distributions are leading to older populations, and the other six regions where the age distributions are younger. These latter countries correspond to the low and middle income countries and contain 85% of the world's population.

The United Nations uses the terms 'developed' and 'less developed' or 'developing' to categorise countries into two broad groups which are similar to the two main World Bank groups. This nomenclature, however, assumes a continuum; the 'developing' countries will not necessarily follow the pattern of wealth generation of the small number of 'developed' countries. Other labels include 'North' and 'South', 'First World' and 'Third World' countries, 'industrialised', 'non-industrialised', and 'newly industrialising'. All of these terms are unsatisfactory and simplistic because, within broad groups of countries, there is enormous diversity in social, economic and health characteristics.

The terms 'rich' (or 'wealthy') and 'poor' are perhaps the most helpful because this simple dichotomy emphasises an important basic distinction between countries. Furthermore, it helps to remind us that rich countries have largely achieved and maintained their position at the expense of the poor countries. For these reasons, we have adopted these terms throughout the book.

1.4 The health transition: a critique

1.4.1 What is the 'health transition'?

The health transition is a framework for describing and explaining the spectacular shifts in the patterns and causes of death that have taken place in most countries[12]. Demographers originally used the term 'demographic transition' or 'mortality transition' to describe the change from high fertility and mortality rates in 'traditional' societies to low fertility and mortality rates in 'modern' societies. A broader term, the 'epidemiological transition', was introduced to describe, in addition to mortality, the long-term changes in patterns of sickness and disability that occurred as societies changed their demographic, economic and social structure[13]. 'Health transition' is a more appropriate term because it includes the social and behavioural changes which parallel, and propel, the epidemiological transition[14].

1.4.2 Health transition: periods, pathways and models

The health transition, as originally described, consists of three periods:

- the era of pestilence and famine;
- the era of receding pandemics; and
- the era of non-communicable diseases (originally called 'man-made' or 'degenerative' diseases, and now often called 'chronic' diseases)[13].

The main feature has been the transition from a pattern dominated by infectious diseases with very high mortality, especially at younger ages, to a pattern dominated by non-communicable diseases and injury with lower overall mortality, which peaks at older ages.

In the era of pestilence life expectancy was low, less than 30 years, and probably higher in men than in women. The major causes of death were due to malnutrition, epidemic infectious diseases, and complications of pregnancy and childbirth. In many western countries the second stage of the transition was established early in the eighteenth century[15] and was dominated by infectious diseases and malnutrition; people lived, on average, up to 50 years. In Western Europe this period lasted until the early twentieth century with the influenza pandemic of 1918–20 being the last major pandemic. The era of non-communicable diseases is characterised by low fertility rates, growth of the population, and an increase in the importance of cardiovascular disease and cancer. In this era, life expectancy is greater in women than men, exceeding 55 years, and ultimately reaches over 80 years. These three periods overlap, and progress is not necessarily linear or progressive; nor are mortality declines necessarily associated with improvements in morbidity and disability.

Recently, a fourth phase of the health transition has been proposed in an attempt to account for the resurgence of 'old' infectious diseases and the emergence of new infectious diseases in association with non-communicable diseases[16,17]. Patterns of mortality and morbidity in this fourth stage have been explained largely on the basis of individual lifestyle[17]. This interpretation is seriously flawed because it exaggerates the role of individual determinants of disease, underplays the power of social and economic determinants of epidemics, and leads to victim blaming.

The pathway from high infectious disease mortality rates is highly variable and not all countries have experienced high rates of non-communicable diseases. In North and Western Europe and North America the benefits of the decline in infectious diseases were, in part, offset by rises in cardiovascular disease and cancer death rates. The increase in non-communicable diseases has been less in Japan, China, and Southern European countries, but greater in countries of Eastern and Central Europe. Non-communicable age-specific disease death rates may not necessarily increase in poor countries as economic and social changes occur, although data to substantiate this suggestion are sparse[18].

It is unlikely that the evolution of the health transition in poor countries will simply be a replication of the pattern of the wealthy countries. In some countries, population growth, poverty, environmental degradation, and the 'demographic' trap, may prevent the transition from high mortality and fertility to low mortality and fertility[19]. This outcome is especially likely in sub-Saharan Africa. Even so, it is important to note that most poor people today have lower death rates than wealthy people a century ago[20].

Three models of the transition, depending on the time and rate of change, have been proposed[13]:

- classical or western;
- accelerated (such as occurred in Japan); and
- the delayed or contemporary model which describes the incomplete transition in poor countries.

Other variations on these models have been proposed to account for the rapidity of the decline in mortality rates this century in middle income countries such as Singapore and South Korea[21]. Different transition models can also occur in different populations within a single country. For example, in New Zealand the European population followed the classical model; more recently the Maori population followed the transitional pattern and has, in turn, been followed by the Pacific Islands population[21]. Some middle income countries, such as Mexico, are following the 'prolonged and polarised model' characterised by overlapping stages (for example, the reappearance of infectious diseases such as malaria that had previously been controlled), and by polarisation, that is, an exacerbation of social class inequalities in mortality rates[22].

1.4.3 What propels the health transition?

There are three major forces underlying the health transition:

- the health determinants;
- the demographic; and
- the therapeutic.

The main driving force includes the underlying social, economic, political and cultural factors which determine health and are responsible for, and propel, the health transition. Of major importance has been the attainment of modest levels of per capita income and widespread literacy, especially for women[23]. Some changes, such as urbanisation and the associated changes in behaviour, occur with industrialisation; other changes are superimposed, for example nutritional changes and the increase in cigarette smoking. An increasing frequency of these risk factors in the population leads to increases in age-specific death rates. Also included in this component are the public health interventions which aim to reduce the population's exposure to health hazards, for example, immunisation and public information campaigns are also included in this component.

The demographic component refers to the universal ageing of populations as a result of declining fertility and, to a lesser extent, to declining death rates, particularly in children. The ageing of the population results in the emergence of the non-communicable diseases of adulthood which have a long latent period and become more frequent with increasing age. As populations age, the absolute number of these diseases will inevitably increase, even if the age and cause-specific death rates decline.

The third driving force, the therapeutic component, includes factors that tend to reduce the risk of dying once disease has become established. Effective health services are essential for the achievement of good population health and interact with the independence of women and higher educational levels. The most effective health services are not necessarily those which are technologically advanced, but rather those which are either free or inexpensive and readily accessible. From a historical perspective, this contribution to the health transition has been small because of the ineffectiveness of most medical interventions. The therapeutic component has been of much more importance in poor countries and has contributed to the major decline in child mortality that has taken place in these countries over the last few decades[23].

1.4.4 The health transition: a critique

The health transition is the best framework for describing the changing patterns of mortality. Nevertheless, it is deficient. Firstly, it fails to explain differences in death rates between countries and has limited ability to predict changing patterns of disease with 'modernisation'. The recent deterioration in life expectancy at middle age in some Central and Eastern European countries and the increasing inequalities in health in all countries were not predicted by the health transition theory. By focusing on the important social and economic causes of changing death rates, however, the health transition offers potential for understanding health trends and thus improving health in all countries.

Secondly, as originally formulated, the epidemiological transition theory with its dichotomy of diseases – infectious or non-communicable – ignores the interaction between disease types; nor were violent deaths, either intentional or unintentional, originally considered. The theory does not easily account for the marked declines that have occurred in mortality rates for some major non-communicable diseases, for example heart disease and stroke. Furthermore, there is a tendency to view the health transition in isolation from the momentous social and economic changes that propelled the transition, especially the nineteenth century European version[24].

Further elaboration of the health transition theory is required. Careful reconstruction of national time series cause-specific mortality patterns is a necessary first step; regional patterns also require exploration[15]. The variability of change according to particular historical, regional and cultural contexts would aid detailed explanation and prediction. Unusual countries and regions might shed useful insights, for example, the phosphate rich Island of Nauru with its high non-communicable disease rates, and the oil rich states of the Middle East with their high mortality rates. The central and influential role of individual and community endeavour in propelling the transition and its interaction with structural change, also require investigation[24]. Health transition research has focused largely on mortality differentials in a single society; more explanatory power would result from cross-country comparisons[25]. With further elaboration, testable hypotheses based on the health transition may be developed.

In summary, although the health transition theory is a useful descriptive tool, it remains a blunt instrument with only limited predictive powers. Epidemiologists, among others, face a major challenge in developing the theory so that it becomes a useful and powerful framework for the study of disease and mortality in populations, both from a historical and contemporary perspective.

1.5 Summary

This introductory chapter has set the scene for the rest of the book by introducing various concepts of health and disease and describing the country and population groupings which we concentrate on in the next chapters. The health transition is the best model available for describing broad changes in patterns of fertility and mortality and morbidity. Unfortunately, it requires more elaboration before it will be of much predictive value. The next chapter describes the major historical trends in mortality and summarises the current state of the world's health.

Chapter 1   Key Points

• Operational definitions of health suitable for summarising trends in the
  status of populations are not available.
• Reliable cause-specific death data are available for only a minority of
  countries.
• All categorisations of countries are simplistic and mask great variation
  within groups and countries.
• The health transition theory provides the best framework for describing
  changing patterns of death but its predictive power is weak.

References

1. *World Health Organization Constitution.* Geneva: WHO, 1946.
2. Dubos R. *Mirage of Health.* New York: Harper, 1959.
3. Mossey JM, Shapiro E. Self-rated health: a predictor of mortality among the
   elderly. *Am J Pub Hlth* 1982; **72**:800–8.
4. Lupton D. Is there life after Foucault? Poststructuralism and the health
   social sciences. *Aust J Pub Hlth* 1993; **17**:298–300.
5. Seedhouse D. The way around health economics' dead end. *Hlth Care
   Analysis* 1995; **3**:205–20
6. Murray CJL, Chen LC. In search of a contemporary theory for
   understanding mortality change. *Soc Sci Med* 1993; **36**:143–55.
7. Rifkin SB, Walt G. Why health improves: defining the issues concerning
   'comprehensive primary health care' and 'selective primary health care'. *Soc
   Sci Med* 1986; **6**:559–66.
8. Hahn RA, Eberhardt S. Life expectancy in four U.S. racial/ethnic
   populations: 1990. *Epidemiology* 1995; **6**:350–5.
9. World Health Organization. *World Health Statistics Annual.* Geneva: WHO,
   1993.
10. Murray CJL, Lopez AL, Jamison D. The global burden of disease in 1990:
    summary results, sensitivity analysis and future directions. *Bull WHO* 1994;
    72:495–509.
11. World Development Report, 1993. *Investing in Health: World Development
    Indicators.* New York: Oxford University Press, 1993.
12. Feachem RGA, Kjellstrom T, Murray CJL, Over M, Phillips MA. *The
    Health of Adults in the Developing World.* New York: Oxford University
    Press, 1991.
13. Omran AR. The epidemiologic transition: a theory of the epidemiology of
    population change. *Milbank Mem Fund Q* 1971; **49**:509–38.
14. Caldwell JC. Introductory thoughts on health transition. In: Caldwell J,
    Findley S, Caldwell P, Santow G, Cosford W, Braid J, Broers-Freeman D
    (eds). *What We Know about Health Transition: the Cultural, Social and
    Behavioural Determinants of Health.* Australian National University,
    Canberra: 1990; 1: xi–xiii.
15. Mackenbach JP. The epidemiologic transition theory. *J Epidemiol Comm
    Hlth* 1994; **48**:329–32.

16. Olshansky SJ, Ault AB. The fourth stage of the epidemiologic transition: the age of delayed degenerative diseases. *Milbank Mem Fund Q* 1986; **64**:355–91.
17. Rogers RG, Hackenberg R. Extending epidemiologic transition theory: a new stage. *Soc Biol* 1987; **34**:234–43.
18. Phillips M, Feachem RGA, Murray CJL, Over M, Kjellstrom T. Adult health: a legitmate concern for developing countries. *Am J Pub Hlth* 1993; **83**:1527–30.
19. King M, Elliott C. Legitimate double-think. *Lancet* 1993; **341**:669–72.
20. Kunitz SJ. Explanations and ideologies of mortality patterns. *Pop Dev Review* 1987; **13**:379–408.
21. Pool I. Cross-comparative perspectives on New Zealand's health. In: Spicer J, Trlin A, Walton JA (eds). *Social Dimensions of Health and Disease: New Zealand Perspectives*. Palmerston North: Dunmore Press, 1994.
22. Frenk J, Bobadilla JL, Sepulveda J, Cervantes ML. Health transition in middle-income countries: new challenges for health care. *Hlth Pol Plan* 1989; **4**:29–39.
23. Caldwell JC. Routes to low mortality in poor countries. *Pop Dev Review* 1986; **12**:171–220.
24. Davis P. A sociocultural critique of transition theory. In: Spicer J, Trlin A, Walton JA (eds). *Social Dimensions of Health and Disease: New Zealand Perspectives*. Palmerston North: Dunmore Press, 1994.
25. Caldwell JC. Health transition: the cultural, social and behavioural determinants of health in the Third World. *Soc Sci Med* 1993; **36**:125–35.

2

Global health: past trends and present challenges

2.1 The global picture: measures of progress

Tremendous improvements have occurred in the health of people in the 200 years since the health transition began. One measure of these changes is that most poor people now live longer, on average, than the wealthiest people a century ago. Despite these gains, there remains a tremendous preventable burden of premature death and disease worldwide.

In this chapter we review the major global trends in mortality and summarise the current state of health of the world's population. The health status of four main population groups will be described: children, women of child bearing age, adults and older people. Children are considered because the vast majority of child deaths are still due to preventable infectious diseases, superimposed on a background of poverty and malnutrition. Furthermore, the main focus of international public health, stimulated by UNICEF (United Nations Children's Fund), continues to be on children[1]. The separate consideration of deaths in association with pregnancy and birth (maternal mortality) is justified because of the tremendous global variation in maternal mortality and the fact that the vast majority of these deaths are preventable. Even so, maternal deaths make up only a very small proportion of the total number of deaths worldwide each year despite the great deal of attention that they receive from international aid organisations.

Deaths in adults are important for four reasons. Firstly, adults make up one-half the population of the world and about 70% of all deaths occur in adults; about half of these deaths are undoubtedly premature, that is, before the age of 60 years[2]. Secondly, adult death rates show considerable regional variation[3]. Thirdly, the nature of adult health problems is quite different to those which continue to preoccupy policy makers in poor countries. The major causes of death in adults in all countries are non-communicable

13

diseases and injuries and these conditions do not respond to the same strategies that have been successful in reducing infectious disease death rates. Adult diseases have received attention in wealthy countries, but the problems of adult non-communicable disease and injuries in poor countries have been neglected. A final justification for a focus on adults is the ageing of the population in all countries. This trend is reflected in the changing pattern of diseases worldwide and, in turn, has major implications for health services and societies in general.

2.1.1 Life expectancy

The dramatic reduction in death rates over the last 200 years can be explained by a number of factors. The most important relate to changes in the cultural, social, economic and behavioural determinants of health and, to a lesser extent, to public health interventions; medical interventions explain only a small amount, although they have had more impact over the last few decades, especially in poor countries. The decline in death rates has led to a major improvement in life expectancy. Life expectancy, the simplest measure of the health of a population, is the average number of years of remaining life, and is always an estimate because it is based on the risk of dying at successive ages within the current population; it assumes no change in death rates in the future.

Our hunter-gathering forebears were lucky to live, on average, 25–30 years; over ensuing centuries, the situation improved very slowly[4]. In the first half of the seventeenth century, for example, life expectancy in western Europe was still not much more than about 25 years, regardless of sex and social class. In nineteenth century England and Wales, life expectancy increased by only seven years, from 41 years in 1841 to 48 in 1901 for the total population[5], in contrast to the rapidity of changes in most countries over the last half century. Since 1901, life expectancy at birth in England and Wales has increased by 28 and 30 years in men and women, respectively, a 60% improvement. Worldwide, life expectancy is now greater in women than in men and over the past two decades has increased 20% faster than male life expectancy[6].

There has also been an increase in the average length of remaining life once a person reaches 65 years of age. At this older age, the most rapid improvements have occurred in the last few decades, largely because of the decline in death rates from heart disease and stroke, two of the major causes of death in adults. At this older age, there was little improvement in life expectancy, especially in men, in the first 50 years of this century.

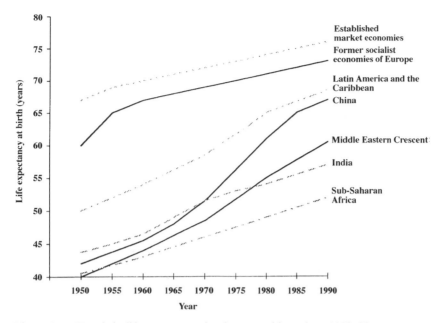

Figure 2.1. Trends in life expectancy by demographic region, 1950–90.
Source: *World Development Report*, 1993 (ref. 2).

Figure 2.1 shows that life expectancy at birth has gradually increased in all regions since 1950[2]. The improvement in China since 1970 is particularly impressive. Even so, the huge disparity between rich and very poor countries has improved very little over the last 40 years. Sub-Saharan Africa showed the slowest improvement in life expectancy in this period, from 39 to 52 years. The contrasting trends in China and India, the two most populous countries, are intriguing and reflect contrasting patterns of social, economic and political development.

The highest life expectancy at birth is now in Japan where boys born in 1993 can expect to live, on average, 76.5 years and girls 83.1 years. There is also a large and increasing difference in life expectancy among the wealthy countries[7]. In some countries of Central and Eastern Europe, life expectancy at birth has been declining over the last decade, indicating that mortality trends are in fact sensitive to countervailing forces[8]. For example, the life expectancy of Russian men in 1995 was only 58 years[9]. An increase in death rates from heart disease, trauma and injury associated with alcohol consumption, and an increase in infant mortality, have all contributed[10]. Some of the fall in life expectancy in Russia may, however, reflect changing registration practices. For example, calculation of infant mortal-

Table 2.1 *Life expectancy, by race/ethnicity and*
gender, United States of America, 1990

	Male (years)	Female (years)
White	72.9	79.4
Asian/Pacific Island	82.0	85.8
American Indian	71.0	78.7
African-American	65.2	73.3

ity rates in Russia did not match the WHO guidelines until 1993; life expectancy in the former Soviet Union may, therefore, have been overestimated. Continuing and worsening economic and industrial disruption in Russia suggest that there is little hope for short-term improvements in Russian vital statistics.

Substantial variations in life expectancy also occur within countries by ethnicity, geographical location and social class. Data from two Dutch villages in the eighteenth century showed that the upper class group had more than a ten-year advantage in life expectancy compared with the lower class group[11]. Relative class inequalities in wealthy countries are still similar to those observed 200 years ago in the Dutch villages[12]. In the United States of America, as shown in Table 2.1, a white male at birth now has a life expectancy, after adjusting for census undercount and misclassification on death certificates, almost eight years greater than that of a male African-American[13].

2.1.2 Fifty million deaths worldwide

There are approximately 50 million deaths worldwide each year, over half of which occur in people less than 60 years of age,[2,14,15]. Table 2.2 shows the distribution of these deaths by country group in four age bands[2]. Four out of five deaths occur in poor countries. Most deaths (50% of the total) occur in adults in poor countries; 25% of all deaths occur in children under five years of age, 99% of these deaths are in poor countries.

The distribution of the 50 million deaths estimated to have occurred in 1993 by broad cause of death is shown in Figure 2.2[14]. Overall 32% of deaths are due to communicable diseases (infectious and parasitic diseases) with another 16% being of unknown cause; over 37% of deaths are due to non-communicable diseases. Injuries are responsible for 8% of deaths globally.

There are striking differences in the pattern of death between the

Table 2.2 *Estimated deaths (in millions) by age, gender and country group, 1993*

Age (years)	Wealthy countries		Poor countries		Total	(%)
	Male	Female	Male	Female		
0–4	0.10	0.09	6.5	6.0	12.6	(25)
5–14	0.03	0.02	1.2	1.1	2.3	(5)
15–59	1.40	0.60	5.6	4.2	11.9	(24)
60 +	4.00	4.60	7.6	7.0	23.2	(46)
Total	5.53	5.31	20.9	18.3	50.0	(100)

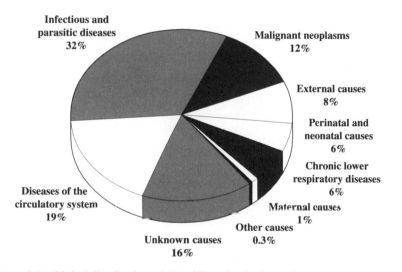

Figure 2.2. Global distribution of 50 million deaths, by main causes. Source: WHO (ref. 14).

wealthy and poor regions as shown in Figure 2.3[14]. Differences in age structure and cause specific death rates account for the varying patterns of death. Communicable diseases are responsible for over 40% of the deaths in poor regions, but for only 1% in wealthy regions. Even in the poor regions, non-communicable diseases account for about one-quarter of all deaths.

The large majority of deaths in wealthy countries are due to non-communicable diseases in adults. For example, of the total of 11 million deaths that occur in wealthy countries, cardiovascular diseases account for 5.5 million a year (half from ischaemic heart disease and a quarter from

Global health

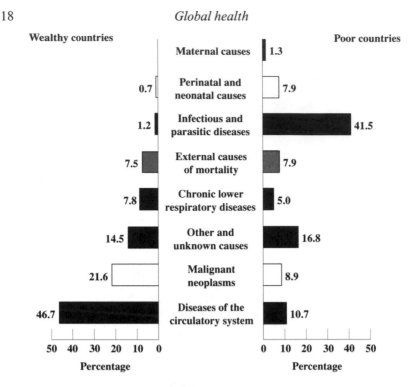

Wealthy countries

Poor countries

Cause	Wealthy	Poor
Maternal causes		1.3
Perinatal and neonatal causes	0.7	7.9
Infectious and parasitic diseases	1.2	41.5
External causes of mortality	7.5	7.9
Chronic lower respiratory diseases	7.8	5.0
Other and unknown causes	14.5	16.8
Malignant neoplasms	21.6	8.9
Diseases of the circulatory system	46.7	10.7

50 40 30 20 10 0   0 10 20 30 40 50
Percentage   Percentage

Figure 2.3. Causes of death in wealthy and poor countries, 1993.
Source: WHO (ref. 14).

stroke), and cancer accounts for another 2.5 million (half a million from lung cancer plus a quarter of a million from other tobacco-caused cancers). The most important remaining cause of death in wealthy countries is respiratory disease which causes just under one million deaths, mostly from chronic obstructive respiratory disease.

2.2 Child deaths

2.2.1 Past trends

The main reason for the universal increase in life expectancy at birth is the improvement in infant and child death rates. These gains have been impressive. In poor agrarian societies last century only one out of two babies survived to the age of 15 years[4]. Infant death in the first year of life (infant mortality) is now a rare event in many countries, occurring only about six times in every 1000 births in countries with the lowest rates. In contrast, in countries with the highest rates, as many as one in eight babies still die in

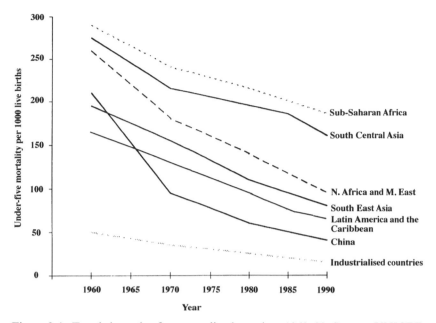

Figure 2.4. Trends in under-five mortality, by region, 1960–90. Source: UNICEF (ref. 22).

the first year of life. Since 1980, increased basic immunisation coverage has saved the lives of about 20 million children[16].

Infant mortality rates are falling slowly in most countries, but the degree of variation between countries has increased over the last 30 years[17]. In 1966, infant mortality was about five times higher in the poorest countries compared with wealthy industrialised countries. In 1992, this ratio had increased to a 12-fold difference[18]. This adverse trend occurred despite international aid and effort and suggests the need for a fundamental restructuring of international and national economic and political relationships, in the interests of the many rather than the few[19].

Death rates in children in the first five years of life (child death rates), are more reliable for regional comparisons because good methods exist for estimating child death rates on the basis of population surveys. Progress has been made in all regions in reducing death rates (Figure 2.4). As with infant mortality rates, however, there has been a worsening of the relative gap between rich and poor countries. For example, in 1960, there was a six-fold variation in child mortality rates between wealthy industrialised countries and sub-Saharan Africa, the region with the highest child mortality rates; by 1992, there was a 16-fold variation. Improvements occurred in sub-Saharan

Africa during the 1950s and 1960s, but since 1970 the rate of progress has slowed[20]. In countries that have recently experienced civil wars such as Somalia, Rwanda, Zaire and the former republics of Yugoslavia, child mortality rates have deteriorated. These wars have claimed the lives of two million children in the past 10 years and left four to five million others crippled for life[16].

2.2.2 *The present*

Globally, approximately 145 million children are born each year with almost 90% of these births occurring in poor countries. In 1993 there were about 12 million deaths in children under five years of age in poor countries of the world[14]. If these children had the same death rate as children in Japan or in the United States of America, there would have been 11.6 million fewer child deaths in 1993.

In poor countries children still die of the infectious diseases that have plagued populations for centuries since the beginning of large settlements[21]. Over 60% of the deaths in children under five years are accounted for by just three broad causes: vaccine preventable diseases (three million), diarrhoea (2.7 million) and respiratory infection (1.7 million)[14]. These infectious disease deaths are the direct result of poverty, malnutrition and low birth weight as well as the absence of comprehensive health services. The vast majority of these deaths can be prevented, often at very low cost, by a combination of social and health policy measures and public health and medical interventions.

At the United Nations World Summit for Children in 1990 most of the world's political leaders agreed upon child health goals for the year 2000. The major goal is for a one-third reduction in under five death rates (or a reduction to 80 per 1000 live births, whichever is lower). Other general goals deal with maternal mortality, malnutrition, safe water, sanitation, education and literacy. Specific goals relate to the protection of children in time of war, protection of girls and women, nutrition and education. Goals for reductions in the common causes of death in childhood were also proposed[22]. Substantial progress is being made in many countries with immunisation coverage, measles reduction, polio eradication, elimination of iodine deficiency, breast feeding, the control of guinea worm, and the provision of safe water and sanitation. Many countries, however, will not meet these targets and, although the Summit Declaration is inspiring, too often the fine words are too often ignored, especially in time of war.

Measles is an example of progress that has been made in reducing infectious disease death rates in children in poor countries. Measles, a relatively mild disease for a healthy child, can be devastating in poor communities. Although the official number of deaths vary and mapping precise trends is impossible, there are now almost 1.5 million fewer deaths each year from measles than occurred in 1980. Unfortunately, the goal of controlling measles by the year 2000, specifically a 90% reduction in cases and a 95% reduction in deaths compared with preimmunisation levels, will not be met in many poor countries. The cornerstone of WHO's measles control policy has been the achievement of a high level of population coverage with measles vaccine; this has not been feasible in many poor countries. Additional strategies have now been developed, including the identification and immunisation of high-risk areas and groups, such as children in poor urban areas and refugees, and the use of selective mass campaigns.

The successes in controlling polio are due to improvements in both childhood nutrition and immunisation campaigns, with half the poor countries reaching the internationally agreed target of 80% coverage for the major vaccine preventable diseases of childhood[18]. Global eradication of polio is far from assured[23], however, and progress is dependent on adequate resources being made available. Oral rehydration therapy for diarrhoea in children is saving over one million child lives a year[18], although in some countries the medical profession is a major stumbling block, preferring drug therapy as a first choice treatment.

Infectious disease deaths still occur in wealthy countries, particularly in marginalised populations. These deaths have been largely prevented in wealthy countries because poverty and malnutrition are much less common and less severe, and preventive child health services are effective. Among wealthy countries there is a five-fold variation in child death rates, from a high in 1992 of 32 per 1000 children in the Russian Federation to a low of six per 1000 children in Japan. This variation is, however, not as great as among poor countries, where the range is almost ten-fold.

In wealthy countries child mortality is dominated by sudden infant death syndrome, congenital disorders and injuries (mostly unintentional). Even these are increasingly preventable; for example, sudden infant death rates have declined dramatically in several countries over a short period as a result of epidemiological research and public health campaigns. Congenital defects show marked social class gradients indicating the importance of environmental factors and the potential for preventive strategies.

2.3 Maternal deaths

2.3.1 Past trends

Maternal mortality rates have improved dramatically over the last two centuries. In Sweden, for example, the rate declined continuously from 1750, with a tremendous improvement occurring in the first 100 years when maternal mortality rates halved from about 1000 per 100000 births to about 500 in the 1850s[24]. Unfortunately, only a few countries have kept such useful long-term population records. An important challenge for epidemiology is the development, maintenance and extension of this type of data.

In the 1880s maternal mortality rates in Western European countries were at least 500 per 100000 births. Rates fell markedly between 1880 and 1910 in Scandinavian countries, but in most other countries they remained high until the 1930s. Since then, reform of obstetric practice, in particular concern about puerperal sepsis, led to a rapid decline in mortality rates. Marked country differences still remain, however. For example, there was a threefold variation among wealthy countries in the late 1980s from a low in Greece to a high in Hungary. Romania has been the exception among the relatively wealthy countries. When abortion and contraception were banned in 1966, maternal mortality rose 40% within five years. By 1989, it was ten times higher than the rate of any other European country. Following the legalisation of abortion in Romania in 1990, the maternal mortality rate fell to 40% of the 1989 level within one year[2].

2.3.2 The present

It might be expected that the measurement of maternal mortality in the 1990s would be easy, but the reality is different. Maternal mortality includes causes of death directly attributable to pregnancy, deaths caused by pre-existing conditions, and deaths due to causes unrelated to the pregnancy. The official definition excludes incidental causes but in practice this does not always occur. Several methods exist to estimate the likely number of maternal deaths but, as with all global health estimates, considerable uncertainty remains. In most of the world, maternal mortality is underestimated because of the absence of an adequate vital registration system. There have been few population based studies of the causes of maternal mortality in poor countries and this hampers an understanding of the real situation[25].

Worldwide about 1% of all deaths occur as a result of the complications of pregnancy. The vast majority, about 500000, occur in poor countries, compared with only 4000 in wealthy countries[14]. The main cause of maternal mortality worldwide is unsafe abortion, responsible for about half of all deaths[26].

The global variation in maternal death rates is greater than for any other population subgroup. The highest maternal mortality rates are in sub-Saharan Africa, where over 700 mothers die for every 100000 births and where the lifetime risk of maternal death is about 1 in 20. By contrast, in Western Europe less than ten mothers die for every 100000 births and the lifetime risk of a maternal death is about 1 in 10000. In the poor countries of the world as a whole, nearly 1 in 200 pregnancies results in the death of the mother, a maternal mortality rate of 450 per 100000 live births. In cases where there is no care or only unskilled care available, as many as one in every 75 pregnancies results in the death of the mother[27]. Young adolescents in Africa and Asia receiving no prenatal care have up to a 5% chance of dying during pregnancy.

The 1990 World Summit for Children goal for maternal mortality was a halving of maternal mortality rates by the year 2000[18]. Achievement of this goal would imply an average maternal mortality rate of 150 deaths per 100000 live births, a level already achieved by several of the poorer countries in the world, for example China and Sri Lanka. This goal is unlikely to be met in much of sub-Saharan Africa without major action for the provision of expanded family planning services and screening, referral, and improved services for antenatal and obstetric care. The challenge is to implement what is already known.

Other important effects of childbirth, apart from maternal mortality, are the morbidity and long-term disability that can result. For example, it has been estimated that there are over 100 acute morbidity episodes for every maternal death. An estimated 62 million women suffer maternal problems annually worldwide with 54 million of these women living in poor countries, 23 million of whom require higher level care for severe complications[28].

2.4 Adult deaths

2.4.1 Past trends

Attention is slowly turning to the marked regional and country variations in adult mortality. As with child and infant mortality, adult mortality has improved, although differences between countries remain great. Figure 2.5

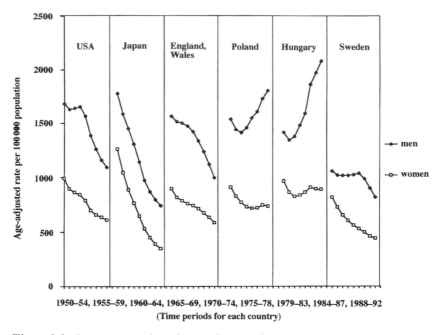

Figure 2.5. Average annual total mortality rates in six selected countries, ages 40–69 years, 1950–90. Men (■), women (□). Source: Thom TJ, *et al.* (ref. 29).

shows trends in adult mortality (people aged 40–69 years) for six wealthy countries for the period 1950–1992[29].

Most countries experienced a fall in total mortality in both men and women over the 40 year period although death rates increased, especially in men, in Central and Eastern Europe. The greatest improvements occurred in Japan; and by the 1980s Japan had the lowest total mortality rates in both men and women. There is still more than a twofold difference between the country with the highest rate (Hungary) and the country with the lowest rate (Japan) in both men and women.

The situation in at least some poor countries is also improving, although reliable data are available for only a few such countries, for example Sri Lanka, Chile, Costa Rica and Cuba. In all four countries, the chances of dying have fallen consistently since the 1950s, except for men in Sri Lanka[30].

2.4.2 The present

The chance of an adult dying prematurely (arbitrarily defined as between the age of 15 and 60 years) varies about tenfold among countries: from more than 50% in parts of sub-Saharan Africa to about 5% in Switzerland and Japan. Among wealthy countries, there is greater variation in adult deaths, especially for men, than in child deaths.

During adulthood differences in the risk of death between regions are largely explained by variations in non-communicable disease death rates, although maternal and communicable deaths remain important in sub-Saharan Africa, and to a lesser extent, in India[31]. Injuries are an important cause of death in men in all regions (one-quarter of all deaths in men aged 15–59 years) and the risk of dying from injury is especially high in Central and Eastern European countries (one-third of all deaths in this age group). It is perhaps surprising that the risk of premature death in men and women from non-communicable diseases is higher in poor countries than in the wealthy countries, apart from Central and Eastern European countries[31].

About ten million premature adult deaths occur each year in poor countries. Non-communicable diseases are the major cause of death in this age group, responsible for half of all deaths. Only one in five deaths in men and one in three deaths in women are due to communicable diseases (including maternal and perinatal causes). Tuberculosis claimed approximately three million deaths in 1995, more than at any time in history[15]. Although the elimination of tuberculosis from human society is a theoretical possibility, there are major impediments to this goal[32].

Even within wealthy countries there are striking variations between ethnic and cultural groups. For example, in the United States of America premature mortality in African-American men and women is 90% and 79% higher than in white men and women, respectively. The death experience of African-American men in the United States is comparable to that among men in some of the poorest nations in the world, such as Gambia and India[31].

The assessment of the relative importance of cause of death depends upon the indicator used. Ranking of causes of death, and the potential years of life lost from a specific cause of death are two useful indicators. In poor countries, the leading causes of deaths for adult women are cardiovascular diseases, cancer, tuberculosis, digestive diseases and respiratory infections; maternal mortality is also important. For men, the ranking is cardiovascular diseases, digestive diseases, unintentional injuries, tuberculosis, cancer and respiratory infections. When potential years of life lost before age 65 years is used as the indicator, conditions that affect younger adults assume greater importance, for example, injuries, tuberculosis and maternal mortality.

The leading causes of death in adults in wealthy countries have not changed substantially since the non-communicable disease epidemics emerged over 70 years ago. The major causes of death account for over half of all adult mortality in the wealthy countries: cardiovascular diseases (coronary heart disease, stroke) and cancer (principally lung cancer in men and women, and breast cancer in women). As cardiovascular disease mortality rates have declined, the proportion of deaths due to cancer has increased and now exceeds the proportion due to coronary heart disease in many wealthy countries. In terms of potential years of life lost in adults in wealthy countries before age 65 years, unintentional injuries are as important as cardiovascular disease and all cancers.

2.4.3 Deaths in older people

As longevity increases in all countries, the health experience of elderly people assumes greater importance, both socially and economically. In 1950 there were approximately 200 million people aged 60 years and over, or 8% of the total population of the world. In 1990, 9.2% of the world's population was over this age and projections suggest that by 2025, the world's elderly population will be around 1.2 billion (or 14% of the total) with the bulk of this increase occurring in poor countries[33] (Figure 2.6). This represents a fourfold expansion in just a quarter of a century.

The rapidity of ageing is without precedent; for example, it took only one-quarter of a century (since 1970) for the proportion of the population 65 years and over in Japan to double (from 7 to 14%). This is in stark contrast to some European countries where the comparative change occurred over a period of 80 to 115 years. It is essential that ageing worldwide be taken seriously in terms of both research and the development of appropriate health and social policies.

The proportion of people 60 years and over in 1990 was higher in wealthy countries (17.7%) than in poor countries (6.9%). More older people live in poor countries, about 285 million people, in contrast to the 202 million people in this age group in wealthy countries. China and India alone have approximately 160 million people over 60 years of age, 27% of all people over this age alive today[31].

Almost a half (46%) of all deaths worldwide occur in people 60 years and over though the proportions differ according to gender (41% of all male deaths and 49% of all deaths in women), and by region (80% of all deaths in wealthy countries and 37% of all deaths in poor countries)[31]. In this older age group, there are 14 million deaths each year in poor regions; the majority, as in wealthy regions, are from non-communicable diseases.

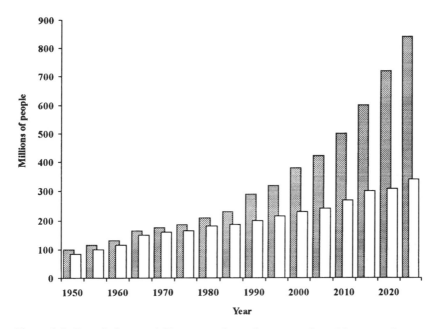

Figure 2.6. Population aged 60 years and over in poor and wealthy countries, 1950–2025. Poor countries (▓); wealthy countries (□). Source: Department of International Economic and Social Affairs (ref. 33).

2.4.4 *Recent trends in causes of adult deaths in wealthy countries*

In the early years of this century, infectious diseases such as tuberculosis were still the leading causes of adult mortality. From about the 1920s, heart disease and stroke became increasingly important, especially in men, along with several kinds of cancer, notably lung cancer. A feature of the trends in the United States of America and many other wealthy countries, is the recent decline in cardiovascular death rates. The greatest decline in cause-specific death rates has occurred in Japan where stroke death rates have declined by about 70% in the last two decades. This illustrates the point that non-communicable disease death rates do not always increase as the health transition occurs; stomach cancer rates have also fallen and coronary heart disease death rates are low in Japan. It remains to be seen whether heart disease rates will stay low in Japan because the diet is slowly changing in an adverse direction, and cigarette smoking is common, especially in men.

There have been several major exceptions to the recent favourable trends in adult mortality patterns, for example AIDS and deaths due to injury. The most notable and longstanding exception, and numerically the most important, however, has been the emergence over the last 50 years of the

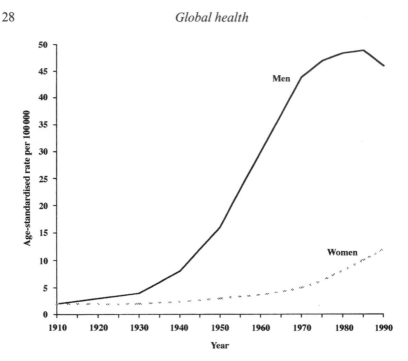

Figure 2.7. Age-standardised mortality rates from lung cancer in men and women, Australia, 1910–14 to 1985–89. Source: Giles GG, *et al.* (ref. 34).

tobacco-caused epidemics, particularly lung cancer. In some countries, such as the United Kingdom, the United States of America and Australia, the lung cancer epidemic has peaked in men, but is still increasing in women. Figure 2.7 shows the age standardised death rates of lung cancer in Australian men and women for the period 1910–14 to 1985–89[34]. The recent age specific trends show greater falls in younger men than in older men.

When the substantial effects of tobacco are discounted, there is little evidence that the overall incidence of cancer is rising[35]. Some cancers, for example, stomach cancer, are declining rapidly, perhaps as a result of dietary changes[36]. It appears that in the United Kingdom, the United States of America and Sweden, rates of some non-smoking-caused cancers may be increasing, for example testicular cancer, melanoma and oesophageal cancer[37]. These trends are important. Although tobacco smoking is the most important preventable cause of cancer and several other diseases, about 70% of cancer cases are not directly linked to smoking; other important environmental causes of cancer remain to be discovered. In many countries, particularly the poorer countries, the tobacco related epidemic is only just beginning, as it takes approximately 20 years of heavy smoking before lung cancer appears.

2.4.5 Recent trends in causes of adult deaths in poor countries

The adult health situation in poor countries is much less clear[30]. The major reason for this uncertainty is the lack of routine cause specific mortality statistics; very few poor countries have 100% medical certification of death[38]. A few countries, such as Singapore which only a few decades ago was considered a poor country, provide excellent mortality data. In Singapore, tuberculosis was the leading cause of death in 1948; since then there has been a rapid increase in the rates of cardiovascular diseases which peaked in the early 1980s, at least in middle-aged people[39].

For most poor countries, indirect methods are required to estimate trends for specific causes of death. The two most populous countries in the world, China and India, have only recently begun to systematically collect mortality data and only for samples of the population. For example, routinely collected data are available for about 100 million people in the eastern provinces of China. The major gap in mortality data is the sub-Saharan African region where no country has the necessary empirical data required for estimating mortality rates for specific causes of death.

Trends in cause specific death rates of adults in poor countries are variable. Some countries such as Chile and Costa Rica have experienced recent increases in life expectancy, and there has been an apparent decline in death rates for the major causes of death[30]. These declines in non-communicable disease death rates are surprising and would not have been predicted on the basis of the health transition as two forces underlying the transition, the demographic and health determinants components, have been acting to increase the age-specific rates of non-communicable diseases. It is extremely unlikely that the health care component is sufficiently powerful to control the increase in the mortality rates. In Cuba, there has been an increase in non-communicable disease death rates, especially in men. In most poor countries, death rates from injury have increased in men. Even if the age-specific rates are declining in some poor countries, the total burden of non-communicable disease in these countries will increase with the ageing of the population. Interpretation of adult mortality trends in poor countries must be cautious until more reliable data are available.

2.4.6 Avoidable deaths

Several estimates have been made of the proportion of deaths which are either avoidable (preventable) or amenable to the effects of health services. One method uses current knowledge to determine the proportion of deaths from each disease which is considered preventable. Another uses as a reference population, a country or population subgroup with low mortality and takes this experience as an ultimately achievable goal for all countries. In this latter method, potentially preventable deaths are those which would not have occurred if the death rates were the same as in the reference population. This method is based on actual death rates and therefore most appropriately reflects what is achievable. Using Japan as the reference population, over 90% of deaths in children less than five years and over 70% of adult deaths in the age group 15–59 years in poor countries are avoidable[2]. Even among older people, there is much room for improvement. For example, in wealthy countries it has been estimated that about one in five of all deaths in men and one in 12 of all deaths in women in the age group 70 years and over are directly related to cigarette smoking[35].

Achieving such major reductions in death rates will not be easy. Indeed, some might consider it an impossible goal. In view of the tremendous reductions in death rates that have occurred in Japan in the last half century, however, cautious optimism is appropriate. Reducing death rates globally to the Japanese level will require a range of policy measures; there is no simple 'magic bullet' intervention. Unfortunately, the improvements in mortality in Japan are not readily explainable, although it does appear that the Japanese commitment to relative income equality has been one factor in their success[40]. Above all, political will is now required to make reducing death rates a global and national priority.

2.5 Disease and disability

2.5.1 Measuring the impact of disease and disability

Premature deaths, because of the great potential for prevention they represent, are a most important challenge for public health. Death alone as an indicator of health status, however, fails to account for the full burden of disease and disability. Various attempts have been made to develop more comprehensive health indicators including a recent estimate of the global burden of disease by the World Bank[2]. The World Bank method combined losses from premature death with the loss of healthy life resulting from disability to calculate the Disability Adjusted Life Years (DALYs) lost for 1990[2]. The total DALYs across all ages, conditions and regions is called the global burden of disease. It measures the present value of the future stream of disability-free life lost because of death, disease or injury in 1990. It is based on events that occurred in 1990 but includes the loss of disability-free life in future years. Several countries are currently measuring trends in DALYs over time to explore its utility for assessing trends in health status and ordering health priorities.

The method of calculating DALYs has many limitations and involves multiple assumptions. In particular, in some regions and for many diseases the necessary data on disease incidence and duration are simply not available. This gap is especially apparent for the adult diseases, which, as we have seen, make up the bulk of the deaths worldwide. For more precise estimates, data are required for subgroups of disease. Furthermore, the method summarises the disease experience on a regional basis, often without any assurance that the data are applicable to the entire region. The data on disability is particularly poor, apart from a few diseases, for example stroke, which have been extensively studied in wealthy countries. Even for stroke, there is a real problem in differentiating stroke related disability from generalised disability. This is an important limitation of the DALYs measure because disability contributes as much as half of all DALYs. Further weaknesses of the global burden of disease estimates concern the subjective assumptions made about disability weights, age weights and discounting weights. It is, however, reassuring that a sensitivity analysis has shown that the results of the global burden of disease study are remarkably insensitive to the particular social preferences incorporated into the calculation of DALYs[41].

Doubts remain about the accuracy of estimates of the global burden of disease. This state has arisen because of the failure of epidemiology to develop the necessary measurement tools. One positive result of the global burden of disease estimates is the identification of basic data needs. Resources are now necessary to ensure that future global burden of disease estimates, and their policy implications, rest on more secure foundations.

2.5.2 *The global burden of disability*

So what does this first attempt at estimating the global burden of disability tell us? Worldwide, an estimated 1.3 billion DALYs were lost in 1990. This is the equivalent of 42 million deaths of new born children or of 80 million deaths at age 50 years. Premature mortality was responsible for 60% of the DALYs lost and disability for the remaining 40%. In the poor world, two-thirds of all DALYs lost were a result of premature mortality compared with just over one-half in rich countries (Figure 2.8)[2].

For the world as a whole, 259 DALYs are lost per 1000 population. There are wide variations among regions. Sub-Saharan Africa loses more than

Global health

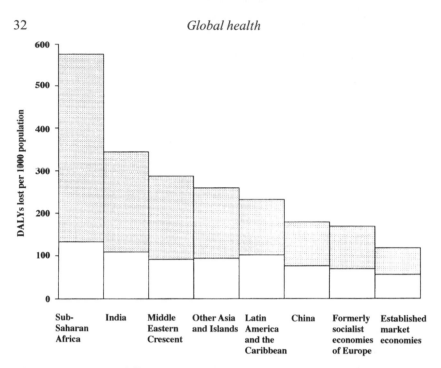

Figure 2.8. Burden of disease (disability adjusted life years: DALYs) attributable to premature mortality and disability, by demographic region, 1990. Disability (□); premature mortality (▨). Source: World Development Report, 1993 (ref. 2).

twice the world average. In wealthy countries the loss is less than half the world average. Most of the difference between regions is due to differences in premature mortality; disability rates are more equal across regions.

Overall, women have about a 10% lower burden of disease per 1000 population than men. Women lose fewer DALYs from premature death, although their DALYs loss from disabilities is overall about the same as for men (Table 2.3)[2]. The female disease burden advantage is more than 30% in the Central and Eastern European countries. Both China and India show a female disadvantage in disease burden. Both countries also have many 'missing' (and presumed dead) women in relation to the expected population balance between the sexes. Foetal screening, followed by sex-selective abortion and female infanticide, account for at least some of the missing women[42].

There is still a tremendous burden of disease due to the preventable and readily curable diseases. One-quarter of the total global burden of disease is accounted for by the childhood epidemic diseases of measles, respiratory infections, worm infections and malaria. The burden of these diseases in

Table 2.3 *Burden of disease by cause and type of loss, 1990*
(millions of DALYs)

Sex and outcome	Disease category		
	Communicable[a]	Non-communicable	Injuries
Men			
Premature death	259	152	72
Disability	47	146	39
Women			
Premature death	244	135	33
Disability	74	142	20

[a] *Includes maternal and perinatal causes* (ref. 2)

children is far larger in sub-Saharan Africa than any other region. Even in adults, communicable diseases continue to contribute significantly to the global burden; sexually transmitted diseases and tuberculosis together, for example, contribute 7% of the global burden of disease.

The higher the disease burden, the higher the proportion attributable to the communicable diseases including maternal and perinatal causes. Non-communicable diseases show the opposite pattern, accounting for 19% of the total burden in sub-Saharan Africa, 43% in Latin America and 78% in the high income countries. Despite this marked difference, the actual rates of loss for both groups of diseases are highest in sub-Saharan Africa and lowest in the wealthiest countries. As health improves, the pattern of disease burden changes; the burden from all types of disease declines and the distribution shifts from communicable to non-communicable disease: the health transition in action.

Despite their shortcomings, the global burden of disease estimates are useful in showing the large burden of premature mortality and disability, particularly in the poorer regions. There are inexpensive and effective ways to dramatically reduce the burden of disease caused by communicable disease which accounts for roughly 35% of the world burden of disease. The reduction of the remaining 65% of the global burden of disease requires other, more complex policy approaches. It remains to be seen, however, whether the global burden of disease estimates are of use to either international aid agencies or national governments in implementing appropriate health programmes.

2.5.3 The impact of disability

Disability is an important component of ill health and a major barrier to human development but its measurement presents enormous difficulties. WHO estimates that globally over 500 million people have an impairment or disability, although disability prevalence rates vary widely[43].

The relationship between mortality and morbidity and disability trends is of considerable importance from a health and social policy perspective. Ideally mortality declines would be accompanied by parallel declines in morbidity. In the 'compression of morbidity' scenario, death is increasingly concentrated at the very oldest ages and occurs in the absence of prolonged sickness and the extra life expectancy gained is free of disease disability[44].

Where life expectancy is increasing, repeated assessments of disability free life expectancy (DFLE) are necessary to determine the quality of the extra years of life. DFLE, a modification of life expectancy, accounts for the proportion of life spent free of disability and is therefore an attempt to capture an aspect of quality of life not addressed by mortality. This indicator was developed over 30 years ago but has only become widely known since the development of the United Nations Disability Statistics Data Base. In comparison with the DALY measure, DFLE is a more objective indicator of the disability process as it does not require the application of weights based on 'expert' opinion. Unfortunately few countries have conducted disability surveys consistently over time.

Disability is difficult to measure and comparisons of DFLEs must be interpreted with caution. Computation of DFLEs from 32 countries, both rich and poor, have now been published in the Statistical World Year Book[45]. Even though life expectancy at birth is similar within a two year span, the DFLEs show greater variation (about eight years) with the differences being consistent for both men and women. As an indicator of relative longevity, the ratio of DFLE to LE (or the percent of total life spent free of disability) can be used to compare countries where life expectancy differs substantially[45].

There are also important gender differences when measuring the impact of disability. For example, 80% of Australian women live to 70 years of age, but only half do so without some measure of disability and a greater number of years lived by women are in a state of severe handicap, when compared with men[46]. A Canadian study suggests that three and a half compromised years are added for each active functional year gained[47] indicating that women pay an increasingly higher price for their longevity; once impaired they will spend a longer time in a disabled state.

The inclusion of disability and its relationships with mortality and morbidity are potentially important contributions to the health transition model discussed in Chapter 1. It is likely that there is also a disability transition that occurs within the health transition as shown in Box 2.1[48].

Box 2.1   Disability in the health transition

It has been hypothesised that during the transition:

- Overall levels of disability incidence are higher in the initial stages of an epidemiological transition and prevalence levels are lower. As the transition proceeds, a reversal of these levels occurs.
- Underlying causes of disablement will shift from those attributable to communicable diseases to non-communicable diseases.
- Disability prevalence levels will shift from being higher at younger ages to being higher at older ages.
- Overall disability will rise with age and disability onset will become more compressed around the average age.
- Prevalence levels of disability will shift from being higher for men to being higher for women.
- Prevalence levels of disability will be greater in lower socioeconomic groups than in higher socioeconomic groups and the differential becomes stronger during the transition.
- Prevalence levels of disablement will increase due to heightened social awareness.
- Healthy life expectancy rises with increasing life expectancy; however, the percentage of life expected to be lived in healthy states declines.

2.6 Inequalities in health

The focus so far in this chapter has been on inequalities in health at the regional level, particularly for conditions that are preventable. Even within countries, major inequalities are apparent and occur irrespective of whether the population is categorised by social class, income, occupation, education or ethnicity. Inequalities in health status have always existed, but it is only over the last few decades, and primarily in the United Kingdom, that social class inequalities have received systematic research attention; epidemiologists usually consider social class as a nuisance variable, rather than as a powerful explanatory variable. The findings from the United Kingdom have now been replicated in most other western countries, although the vital statistics of the United States of America only report basic data about the health of the nation in terms of race, sex, and age[49]. Evidence is also emerging on the existence of health inequalities in Central and Eastern European countries[50].

Entrenched health inequalities reflect the failure of social policy to address social and economic deprivation. Inequalities have also been seen either as a biological phenomenon associated with random variation in the population distribution of health[51], or as the unintended consequences of success in expanding the advantages of the upper social classes[52]. Random variation is an unlikely explanation given that the extent, and even the direction, of health inequalities can change surprisingly quickly[53]. From a human rights perspective, the health of one group of people should not be valued more highly than that of other groups.

Social class patterns have changed over the last 40 years. For example, from the 1930s to the 1950s coronary heart disease rates were highest in the upper social classes in the United Kingdom, but by the 1970s the pattern had reversed[54]. Despite the continuing decline in mortality rates, social class gradients have either remained constant or increased; Japan is an exception in that social class differences in mortality have apparently narrowed since the 1950s[40]. Even within occupational groups which are far from deprived, such as British civil servants, there is a sharp social class effect[55]. This indicates the importance to health of relative deprivation, in addition to the more widely recognised effects of absolute deprivation.

It is more difficult to assess the links between social class and mortality for women than it is for men because of the way social class is usually measured. In most national vital registration systems, a women's position is based on her husband's occupational status; this ignores the independence of a woman's life separate from her spouse[56]. In an attempt to overcome this problem a variety of additional data derived from a British longitudinal study linking census and mortality data have been examined[57]. High mortality rates among women were associated with working in a manual occupation, being a single woman in a manual occupation, living in a rented house, and having no access to a car. When these indicators are combined, mortality rates were found to be two to three times higher than for women with none of these disadvantages[56]. These data indicate that it is necessary to use multiple measures to accurately reflect the relationship between a woman's life circumstances and mortality.

Several possible explanations for the health inequalities have been advanced: misclassification of social class, particularly in women and retired people; a downward drift because of ill health; inequalities in the distribution of major risk factors for disease; generalised susceptibility to ill health in lower social classes; and inequalities in the distribution of income. Epidemiological research allows several of these explanations to be rejected. Misclassification and downward drift can be ruled out on the evidence from long-term epidemiological studies. Inequalities in the distribution of known risk factors for cardiovascular disease or cancer explain only a part of the inequalities in death and disease[55]. An important reason for inequalities in health appears to be the distribution of wealth within a country[58]. In countries where income distribution is relatively equal, health inequalities are less than in countries where there are gross disparities in wealth. This explanation will be explored in more depth in the next chapter. At a more general level, health inequalities reflect social policies which neglect the needs of poor people.

2.7 Explaining trends in mortality

The historical improvements in mortality rates have been obvious and dramatic. We cannot assume, however, that life expectancy will continue to increase into the next century, especially given the experience of some Central and Eastern European countries where life expectancy has fallen dramatically in recent years.

The explanations for these trends are difficult to disentangle and the health transition theory provides only limited guidance. In part, our difficulty stems from the multi-factorial nature of the causes of death. Another problem is our limited ability to relate changes in possible causes and mortality trends at a population level in any meaningful quantitative manner. A further complication stems from the focus on mortality trends in Western Europe, justified on the basis of the availability of better long-term data from this region. The population of Western Europe, however, is only a small (and diminishing) proportion of the world's population. Furthermore, most countries of the world, including the most populous (China and India), have experienced major mortality declines only in the last few decades. The causes of the mortality decline in Western Europe in the nineteenth century will be different from the causes operating in China and India in the late twentieth century.

Various explanations have been advanced for the decline in mortality rates which gathered speed in nineteenth century Europe. McKeown proposed that steady improvements in nutrition beginning in the eighteenth century, together with improvements in water supply and sanitation services, an increase in the general standard of living following the industrial revolution, and a reduction in birth rates propelled the health transition[59]. The development of effective medical measures was too late to make a major contribution to the mortality decline in Europe and other western countries. For example, it has been estimated that at most, only 3.5% of the total decline in mortality in the United States of America between 1900 and 1973 could be ascribed to medical measures introduced for the major infectious diseases[60]. On the other hand, targeted public health interventions including vaccination, personal hygiene campaigns, and improved child health care services, have also been of major importance[4,61].

McKeown's thesis generated controversy which was fuelled by critics of medicine, such as Illich[62], who were concerned at the medicalisation of modern society and the power of the health professionals. Ironically, McKeown's ideas also indirectly encouraged many economists in the belief that improvements in health for the entire population would come from unrestrained economic development and that a reduction in social and health inequalities should not necessarily be a priority of social policy. One unfortunate effect of this policy has been a widening of income inequality. For example, the lowest 10% of the population in the United Kingdom in terms of income are now about 17% worse off than they were in 1979[63].

The more recent decline in mortality in poorer countries has some parallels with nineteenth century Europe. For example, the dramatic gains in China in the last four decades were associated with major improvements in food supply (despite occasional devastating famines) as well as public health campaigns directed at the control of infectious diseases; literacy, especially for females, has also been of major importance[64]. The most recent declines in mortality, however, have been greatly influenced by public health and medical care advances[65]. For example, smallpox, a major scourge of humankind for centuries, has been eradicated, and for a period, malaria was controlled in many parts of the world. And as we have seen, children have benefited from global efforts to increase immunisation coverage, oral rehydration therapy for diarrhoea, and appropriate care for acute respiratory infections.

The modern decline in mortality from non-communicable diseases in rich countries also shows the influence of both public health campaigns and medical care. The major influence in the early stages of the decline in coronary heart disease mortality beginning in the late 1960s, appears to have been changes in diet and smoking habits, although the evidence is incomplete. More recent trends have occurred as a result of major reductions in community risk factor levels, accounting, for example, for much of the decline in coronary heart disease death rates in Finland between 1970 and 1985[66]. Risk factor levels have improved as a result of public health campaigns directed primarily at the population as a whole. Medical care of established cardiovascular disease has been shown to be effective in reducing case fatality, especially in hospitalised patients, but from a population perspective, is making only a small contribution to the mortality declines[67]. In contrast, lung cancer rates are declining in men in some countries purely as a result of public health campaigns, as medical and surgical therapy has little impact on lung cancer death rates.

Evidence from population groups which have undergone the health transition in the last few decades, for example New Zealand Maori, indicate the importance of health policies nested in the context of positive social policies. The New Zealand governments of the early decades of this century, and in particular the Labour Government of 1933–38, implemented a wide range of policies to strengthen the welfare state; collectively these policies had a dramatic and beneficial impact on Maori mortality rates[68].

There are important lessons to be learnt from the health transition in both rich and poor countries. Historically, social and economic developments which improved nutritional status and sanitary systems and increased the literacy of women have been of major importance. General developments have interacted with more specific public health measures directed towards the control of infectious diseases and, more recently, non-communicable disease. Medical care services do have an impact on population mortality trends, especially on child mortality in poor countries; for adults this impact is smaller, although these services are of tremendous importance in relieving suffering. The major gains in health status in the future will come most effectively and efficiently from public health measures.

2.8 Summary

Our attempt to describe worldwide health trends has been severely hampered by the lack of routine health statistics in most countries. There are almost no data available to assess trends using a definition of health which extends beyond mortality. From the data that are available, however, death rates are declining and life expectancy is continuing to increase, except in countries in sub-Saharan Africa and Central and Eastern Europe. Despite these improvements, major inequalities in mortality between regions, and within regions, have remained almost unchanged over the last few decades.

The health transition continues unevenly. In wealthy countries, child and maternal mortality rates are low, and the major causes of adult deaths are cardiovascular diseases which are declining in most countries, and cancer. In poor countries the trends are variable, although statistics are scarce;

however, most poor people today have lower mortality rates than wealthy people a century ago, indicating the important influence of the social, political, and economic environment on health status. Childhood infectious disease death rates have declined, but much preventable infectious disease remains.

The trend data indicate that major improvements in death rates can occur over a relatively short time. The major feature of the current patterns of health worldwide is the enormous variation in the mortality and disease burden, especially between regions and countries, but also within countries. Most of the differences in the burden of disease between regions is due to differences in premature death; disability rates are more equal across regions. Furthermore, most of the regional mortality variations are due to the infectious diseases which are readily preventable. Poor countries experience the greatest burden from non-communicable diseases and these too are largely preventable, although they require more complex strategies than the prevention of infectious diseases.

Chapter 2   Key Points

- Major global improvements have occurred in health status over the last five decades as measured by declining death rates and increasing life expectancy.
- The global inequalities in relative death rates have not changed substantially and death rates have increased recently in some Central and Eastern European countries.
- Detailed cause of death information is available for only one-third of the world's population.
- Of the 50 million deaths each year, half occur before the age of 60 years and 80% occur in poor countries. One-third of deaths are due to communicable diseases and almost half to non-communicable diseases and injuries; the epidemics of non-communicable diseases will inevitably increase as the world's population ages.
- Premature deaths are responsible for about 60% of the Disability Adjusted Life Years lost in 1990; disability was responsible for the remaining 40%.
- Entrenched inequalities in health status exist in all countries.

References

1. Phillips M, Feachem RGA, Murray CJL, Over M, Kjellstrom T. Adult health: a legitimate concern for developing countries. *Am J Pub Hlth* 1993; **83**:1527–30.
2. World Development Report. *Investing in Health: World Development Indicators.* New York: Oxford University Press, 1993.
3. Kitange HM, Machibya H, Black J, Mtasiwa DM, Masuki G, *et al.* Outlook for survivors of childhood in sub-Saharan Africa: adult mortality in Tanzania. *Br Med J* 1996; **312**:216–20.
4. Powles J. Changes in disease patterns and related social trends. *Soc Sci Med* 1992; **35**:377–87.
5. Woods R. The role of public health initiatives in the nineteenth-century mortality decline. In: Caldwell J, Findley S, Caldwell P, Santow G, Cosford W, Braid J, Boers-Freeman D (eds). *What We Know About Health Transition: The Cultural, Social and Behavioural Determinants of Health.* Canberra: Australian National University Printing Service, 1990; 1:110–15.
6. United Nations Development Programme. *Human Development Report 1994.* New York: Oxford University Press, 1994.
7. Bobak M, Marmot M. East-West mortality divide and its potential explanations: proposed research agenda. *Br Med J* 1996; **312**:421–5.
8. Murray CJL, Chen LC. In search of a contemporary theory for understanding mortality change. *Soc Sci Med* 1993; **36**:143–55.
9. Ingram M. Russian life expectancy rises. *Br Med J* 1996; **312**:799.
10. Anon. Life expectancy in Russia falls. *Br Med J* 1994; **308**:4.
11. Schellekens J. Mortality and socioeconomic status in two eighteenth century Dutch villages. *Population Studies* 1989; **43**:391–404.
12. Najman JM. Health and poverty: past, present and prospects for the future. *Soc Sci Med* 1993; **36**:157–66.
13. Hahn RA, Eberhardt S. Life expectancy in four U.S. racial/ethnic populations: 1990. *Epidemiology* 1995; **6**:350–5.
14. World Health Organization. *The World Health Report 1995: Bridging the Gaps.* Geneva: WHO, 1995.
15. World Health Organization. *The World Health Report 1996: Fighting Disease, Fostering Development.* Geneva: WHO, 1996.
16. UNICEF. *The State of the World's Children.* New York: Oxford University Press, 1996.
17. World Health Organization. *World Health Statistics Annual.* Geneva: WHO, 1993.
18. UNICEF. *The State of the World's Children.* New York: Oxford University Press, 1994.
19. UNICEF. *The State of the World's Children.* New York: Oxford University Press, 1995.
20. Feachem RGA, Jamison DT. *Disease and Mortality in Sub-Saharan Africa.* New York: Oxford University Press, 1991.
21. Horton R. The infected metropolis. *Lancet* 1996; **347**:134–5.
22. UNICEF. *The State of the World's Children.* New York: Oxford University Press, 1992.
23. Hull HF, Lee JW. Sabin, Salk or sequential? *Lancet* 1996; **347**:630.
24. Högberg U, Wall S. Secular trends in maternal mortality rates in Sweden, 1750–1980. *Bull WHO* 1986; **64**:79–84.

25. Malcoe LH. National policy, social conditions, and the etiology of maternal mortality. *Epidemiology* 1994; **5**:481–3.
26. Tonks A. Pregnancy's toll in the developing world. *Br Med J* 1994; **108**:353–4.
27. UNICEF *Children and Development in the 1990s.* New York: UNICEF, 1990.
28. Koblinsky MA, Campbell OMR, Harlow S. Mother and more: a broader perspective in women's health. In: Koblinsky MA, Timyan J, Gay J (eds). *The Health of Women: A Global Perspective.* Boulder: Westview Press, 1992.
29. Thom TJ, Epstein FH, Feldman JJ, Leaverton PE, Wolz M (eds). *Total Mortality and Mortality from Heart Disease, Cancer and Stroke from 1950 to 1987 in 27 Countries. Highlights of Trends and their Interrelationships among Causes of Death.* National Institutes of Health: US Department of Health and Human Services, Public Health Service, 1992.
30. Feachem RGA, Kjellstrom T, Murray CJL, Over M, Phillips MA (eds). *The Health of Adults in the Developing World.* New York: Oxford University Press, 1991.
31. Murray CJL, Lopez AL. Global and regional cause of death patterns in 1990. *Bull WHO* 1994; **72**:447–80.
32. Enarson DA. The challenge of tuberculosis: statements on global control and prevention. *Lancet* 1995; **346**:809–10.
33. Department of International Economic and Social Affairs. *Periodical on Aging*, vol, 1, no. 1. New York: United Nations, 1995.
34. Giles GG, Hill DJ, Silver B. The lung cancer epidemic in Australia, 1910–1989. *Aust J Pub Hlth* 1991; **15**:245–7.
35. Peto R, Lopez AD, Boreham J, Thun M, Heath C. *Mortality from Smoking in Developed Countries 1950–2000: indirect Estimates from National Vital Statistics.* Oxford: Oxford University Press, 1994.
36. Coggon D, Inskip H. Is there an epidemic of cancer? *Br Med J* 1994; **308**:705–8.
37. Davis DL, Dinse GE, Hoel DG. Decreasing cardiovascular disease and increasing cancer among whites in the United States from 1973 through 1987: good news and bad news. *JAMA* 1994; **271**:431–7.
38. Lopez AD. Assessing the burden of mortality from cardiovascular disease. *WHO Stat Q* 1993; **46**:91–6.
39. Hughes K. Trends in mortality from ischaemic heart disease in Singapore, 1959 to 1983. *Int J Epidemiol* 1986; **15**:44–50.
40. Marmot MG, Davey-Smith G. Why are the Japanese living longer? *Br Med J* 1989; **299**:1547–51.
41. Murray CJL, Lopez AL, Jamison D. The global burden of disease in 1990: summary results, sensitivity analysis and future directions. *Bull WHO* 1994; **72**:495–509.
42. Anon. Evidence mounts for sex-selective abortion in Asia. *Asia-Pac Pop Pol* 1995; **34**:1–4.
43. Haber LD, Dowd JE. *A Human Development Agenda for Disability: Statistical Considerations.* United Nations Statistical Division of the Department for Economic and Social Information and Policy Analysis. 1994.
44. Fries JF, Green LW, Levine S. Health promotion and the compression of morbidity. *Lancet* 1989; **i**:481–3.
45. REVES. *Supplement to bibliograph Series No 4.* Statistical World Yearbook, Retrospective, 1993.
46. Kinsella K, Taeuber CM. *An Aging World II.* Washington: US Bureau of the Census, US Government Printing Office, 1992.

47. Wilkins R, Adams OB. Health expectancy in Canada, late 1970s: demographic, regional and social dimensions. *Am J Pub Hlth* 1983; **73**:1073–80.
48. Myers GC, Lamb VL. Theoretical perspectives on healthy life expectancy. In: Robine JM, Mathers CD, Bone MR, Romieu I (eds). *INSERM*. John Libbey Eurotext Ltd, 1993.
49. Moss N, Krieger N. Report on the Conference of the National Institutes of Health. *Pub Hlth Reports* 1995; **110**:302–5.
50. Wnuk-Lipinski E, Illsley R. International comparative analysis: main findings and conclusions. *Soc Sci Med* 1990; **31**:879–89.
51. St.Leger AS. Inequalities and health. *Lancet* 1994; **343**:538.
52. Charlton BG. Is inequality bad for the national health? *Lancet* 1994; **343**:221–2.
53. Marmot MG, McDowall ME. Mortality decline and widening social inequalities. *Lancet* 1986; **ii**:274–6.
54. Marmot MG, Adelstein AM, Robinson N, Rose G. Changing social class distribution of heart disease. *Br Med J* 1978; **2**:1109–12.
55. Marmot M. Social differences in mortality: the Whitehall Studies. In: Lopez AD, Caselli G, Valkonen T (eds). *Adult Mortality in Developed Countries: From Description to Explanation*. Oxford: Oxford University Press, 1995.
56. Pugh H, Moser K. Measuring women's mortality differences. In: Roberts H (ed). *Women's Health Counts*. London: Routledge, 1990.
57. Moser KA, Fox AJ, Jones DR. Unemployment and mortality in the OPCS longitudinal study. *Lancet* 1984; **ii**:1324–9.
58. Wilkinson RG. Income distribution and life expectancy. *Br Med J* 1992; **304**:165–8.
59. McKeown T. *The Role of Medicine – Dream, Mirage or Nemesis*. London: Nuffield Provincial Hospitals Trust, 1976.
60. McKinlay JB, McKinlay SM. The questionable effect of medical measures on the decline of mortality in the United States in the twentieth century. *Milbank Mem Fund Q* 1977; **55**:405–28.
61. Szreter S. The importance of social intervention in Britain's mortality decline c. 1850–1914: a re-interpretation of the role of public health. *Society for the Social History of Medicine* 1988; **1**:1–37.
62. Illich I. *Limits of Medicine. Medical Nemesis: The Expropriation of Health*. Harmondsworth: Penguin, 1981.
63. Dean M. Absolute effects of relative poverty. *Lancet* 1994; **344**:463.
64. Caldwell JC. Routes to low mortality in poor countries. *Pop Dev Review* 1986; **12**:171–220.
65. Warren KS. McKeown's mistake. *Health Transition Review* 1991; **1**:229–33.
66. Jousilahti P, Vartiainen E, Tuomilehto J, Pekkanen J, Puska P. Effect of risk factors and changes in risk factors on coronary mortality in three cohorts of middle – aged people in Eastern Finland. *Am J Epidemiol* 1995; **141**:50–60.
67. Beaglehole R, Stewart AW, Jackson R, Dobson A, McElduff P, D'Este K, Heller R, Jamrozik K, Hobbs M, Parsons R, Broadhurst R. Declining rates of coronary heart disease in New Zealand and Australia, 1983–1993. *Am J Epidemiol* 1997; 145: 707–13.
68. Pool I. Cross-comparative perspectives on New Zealand's health. In: Spicer J, Trlin A, Walton JA (eds). *Social Dimensions of Health and Disease: New Zealand Perspectives*. Palmerston North: Dunmore Press, 1994.

3

Contemporary global health issues

3.1 Introduction

The burden of premature death worldwide represents a tremendous challenge to all concerned with public health. The most important causes of ill health are the social and economic characteristics of a society which are the driving force underlying the health transition. Unfortunately, these major determinants are often poorly defined and, from a policy perspective, too often neglected.

The broad definition of the term 'cause' used in this book refers to any factor that directly or indirectly influences health in either direction. Of course, the mere existence of a cause does not necessarily imply that it will lead to a health state or disease. For example, motor vehicles are not inevitably associated with death and destruction; countries with the same number of cars per head of population can have quite different rates of death from car crashes because of different approaches to prevention. In reality it is simplistic to think in terms of single 'causes' of disease. Complex pathways, mechanisms and multiple systems are involved. The evidence on social class gradients suggests, for example, that some underlying causal process associated with social integration may express itself though different diseases[1].

The health status of a population reflects the interaction between its genetic endowment and environmental conditions. There is abundant evidence, however, that the major health and disease differences between populations are caused by environmental rather than genetic factors[2]. For example, the striking international differences in death rates from cardiovascular disease, the rapid changes in these rates over time, and the impact of migration on disease rates, all testify to the importance of the environment in determining the health status of a population. The modification of environmental factors is the most logical and cost effective approach to health improvement. Genetic factors are however, responsible for some of the differences in disease experience within populations. Not all smokers, for example, get lung cancer, suggesting that genetic factors may contribute to this important cause of death and disease, although other environmental factors, such as diet, may also contribute[3]. Within populations it is the way in which an individual's genetic predisposition interacts with other environmental determinants of health that is of critical importance. Until recently, genetic factors have been thought of as being fixed and unchangeable. Now, however, specific genes responsible for some relatively uncommon diseases (such as cystic fibrosis) have been identified. No doubt an increasing number of genes will be found to be associated with specific diseases as a result of the human genome project. Despite the huge cost of this research, it is unlikely, from a global perspective, that major positive health impacts will result from genetic manipulation.

3.2 Underlying socioeconomic causes

3.2.1 Health, wealth and poverty

Important for health, above all else, is a basic level of wealth sufficient to supply essential needs such as food, shelter, clothing and warmth. In traditional societies, wealth was measured in a variety of ways; in most societies wealth is now measured in terms of personal and family income. Inequalities in wealth and power lead to inequalities in health by determining the social circumstances in which people work and live.

Industrialisation, and the wealth it created, has had major and variable impacts on the health of nations. The countries of Europe and North America which industrialised early, ultimately experienced huge overall health benefits, although as we have seen, striking inequalities in health status are entrenched in these countries. Much of the benefit reaped by the wealthy countries has been at the expense of their former colonies which continue to provide a source of cheap labour, resources and open markets. In this sense, wealthy and poor countries, rather than being part of a linear process, act as complementary participants in the overall global process of industrialisation[4].

The relationships between economic development and health are complex. Once a minimum level of per capita income is achieved, social and political priorities have a greater impact on the health status of the population than overall national wealth. This finding is critical and is in contrast to the generally accepted view that the health of a population will improve only as a nation 'develops' and becomes increasingly wealthy. This assumption ignores the evidence that uncontrolled economic growth, which encourages production and consumption, is responsible for much of the global environmental destruction. The main favourable effects of economic growth on health include improvements in nutrition, both in quality and quantity, effective public health measures, medical care, effective birth control, improvements in physical environment, and widespread literacy[5].

Poverty is a striking feature of the world today. The criteria for poverty vary. The World Bank's description of poverty is 'a condition of life so limited by malnutrition, literacy, disease, squalid surroundings, high infant mortality, and low life expectancy as to be beneath any reasonable definition of human decency'; absolute poverty is defined as a per capita annual income of about US$450[6]. Approximately 1.3 billion people are estimated to live in absolute poverty, over 70% of whom are women[7] (Box 3.1).

Box 3.1 Women in poverty[7]

Poverty is the condition of the vast majority of the world's women. Almost two-thirds live in countries classified by the United Nations as having 'very low GDP' (<$1000 per capita). Another 13% live in countries where per capita income, by the UN definition, is 'low' ($1000 to $3000 per capita annually).

In every country, at every socioeconomic level, women control fewer productive assets than do men; they also work longer hours but earn less income. Lacking alternatives, women are more often compelled to resort to jobs that are seasonal, labour intensive and carry considerable occupational risks. Thus poverty for women is more intractable than for men, and their health is even more vulnerable to adverse changes in social and environmental conditions.

Women's work is grossly unpaid, unrecognised, and undervalued to the order of US$11 trillion a year. Yet it has been estimated that the total bill to provide basic services to women in every developing country is around $20 billion a year, or only 5% of the total size of public sector budgets in poor countries.

Poverty and powerlessness, two problems which women suffer disproportionately, are serious health hazards. In no country in the world are women offered the same socioeconomic and political opportunities as men; women lag behind men on virtually every indicator of social and economic status.

Table 3.1 *Poverty in poor regions of the world, 1985–90*

Region	% of the population below the poverty line[a]		Number of poor (millions)	
	1985	1990	1985	1990
South Asia	52	49	532	562
East Asia and Pacific	13	11	182	169
Sub-Saharan Africa	48	48	184	216
Middle East and North Africa	31	33	60	73
Latin America and Caribbean	22	25	87	108

[a] Defined as $31 per person per month at 1985 prices (ref. 8)

Another two billion people have incomes insufficient to meet more than the most basic needs.

Although there have been slight reductions in world poverty in percentage terms, the absolute numbers of poor people increased in the 1980s, especially in the low and middle income countries of South Asia and sub-Saharan Africa. In 1990 almost half the populations of sub-Saharan Africa and South Asia were below the World Bank's poverty line, compared with 7% in eastern Europe (Table 3.1)[8].

The average annual income is around 50 times higher in the rich countries than in the three-fifths of the world's population living in poor countries, and the gap is growing. The total wealth of the world's 358 billionaires equals the combined incomes of the poorest 45% of the world's population[9]. The distribution of wealth within countries is also very uneven. The greatest inequality in income distribution occurs in the poorest countries. For example, there is a 20–30-fold difference between the richest and poorest fifths of the population in Mexico and Brazil[10]. Even in wealthy countries, poverty levels can change surprisingly rapidly. In the United States of America during the 1980s, the richest 1% increased their share of the nation's wealth from around 31 to 37%, yet in 1991, it was estimated that almost one-fifth of total mortality in people aged 25–74 years of age was attributed to poverty[11]. In the United Kingdom there was a threefold increase in the proportion of children living below the European Union's poverty line in the last decade; about one in three children are now below this line[12]. In relatively wealthy countries, the vast majority of those in poverty belong to one of five groups: single parents and their children, the aged, the unemployed, racial and ethnic minorities, and the disabled. Three of these groups (single mothers, the aged and the disabled) are likely to increase in numbers[13].

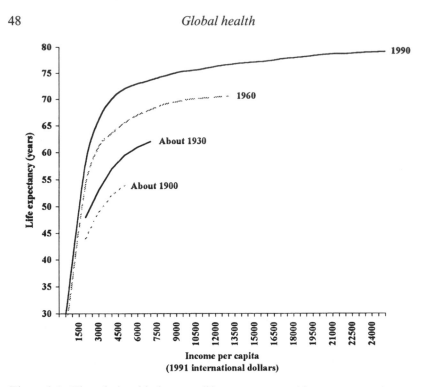

Figure 3.1. The relationship between life expectancy and income per capita.
Source: World Development Report, 1993 (ref. 6).

Health is not a straightforward function of wealth. The complex relationship between life expectancy and income per capita for selected countries and four periods is shown in Figure 3.1[6]. As measured by life
expectancy at birth, health improves rapidly as average per capita
increases up to $5000 (1991 International dollars) per person. A doubling
of income from $1000 in 1990 corresponds to a gain in life expectancy of
about 11 years, whereas a doubling from an income of $4000 would be
associated with a gain of only about four years. Above a mean of about
$5000, per capita income itself is no longer the critical determinant of
health status[14]. The rich Middle Eastern oil producing countries (which
are mainly Moslem) illustrate the complexity of this relationship; life
expectancy in these countries is relatively low. On the other hand, several
countries such as Sri Lanka and China, have much higher levels of life
expectancy than would be expected from their per capita incomes (GNP
per capita in 1992 of less than US$600)[15]. Another clue to the importance
of factors other than income is that, over time, a given level of income has
become associated with a longer life expectancy. For example, in 1900 an

income of $5000 per capita was associated with a life expectancy of about 55 years; in 1990 this income level was associated with a life expectancy of about 70 years.

In general, once countries reach a per capita income of more than $5000, health standards become dependent on the distribution of income and the effectiveness of public policies[16]. Expenditures on health personnel and health facilities explains much less of the variation in life expectancy than social factors such as literacy, nutrition, transportation and communications[17]. Poor countries which have achieved exceptionally high standards of health, for example China and Cuba, demonstrate the importance of female autonomy and literacy and the political will to make health a priority, especially for women and children[18,19].

As income distribution within a country narrows, life expectancy increases[20]. The widening of the income gap between rich and poor in the United Kingdom over recent decades is reflected in a slowdown in the decline in mortality in young people in Britain[12]. Sometimes, seemingly remote policy decisions have an unexpected health impact. For example, the value added tax on fuel in the United Kingdom has increased the overall tax burden unevenly and added to the redistribution of wealth from the poor to the rich[21].

Economic inequality may affect health both directly and indirectly through psychological and social processes, by effects on self-esteem, and on social relations generally[22]. The Japanese workers' advantage over British workers is not due to a greater spending on health care in Japan but may be explained by the fact that material rewards for work are more evenly distributed in Japan[20,23]. In recent decades income distribution in Japan has become the narrowest of any country; very low military expenditure has allowed greater investment in other sectors[24]. At an even more general level, the relative increase in the position of Japan in comparison with other countries may in turn have a positive impact on Japanese self-esteem and thus on health.

Unfortunately, from an epidemiological perspective, the data supporting the association between the distribution of wealth and health are not conclusive. There are many ways in which countries differ, apart from the distribution of wealth. Even within countries the rich differ from the poor in many ways other than income. Furthermore, the health implications of relative deprivation, as opposed to absolute poverty, are also of great importance[25,26]. The profound policy implications of the association of wealth and health make this an essential area for further research.

The immediate cause of poverty of an individual or family is either unemployment or being in underpaid employment. Unemployment has an effect on health directly through poverty but also through other mechanisms involving psychosocial pathways[27]. Poverty is associated with a whole range of adverse health effects. Poor people have less income to spend on nutritious food, clean water, adequate clothing and shelter, all of which are essential to a minimum level of health and well-being. They also have less access to education and political power which is needed to improve and safeguard health. Even limited economic progress in poor countries would have a major beneficial impact on health, so long as the wealth gained is distributed equitably, and so long as the economic progress is sustainable and not at the expense of the environment.

The World Health Organization has identified poverty as 'the greatest single killer'[28]. The alleviation of poverty is the most pressing issue facing public health practitioners and society in general[29]. Not only is this the major immediate global health challenge, it is also necessary for the development of a sustainable global economy. Dealing with this challenge will require skills far beyond those required for the design and implementation of traditional public health programmes. An important first step is recognition of the need, in the interests of health, for income redistribution policies[30]. Economic growth alone is insufficient to overcome absolute poverty and will have little impact on relative poverty[22].

3.2.2 Other socioeconomic causes

Inadequate housing is a major cause of ill health in all countries. Rapid urbanisation is causing a crisis in housing and future prospects look bleak[31]. The urban population in poor countries will almost triple (from 1.4 to 3.8 billion) during the next 30 years while the rural population will increase by about 10%[32]. Most of the new urban residents will live in slums with poor or non-existent health services[33]. Homelessness is also an increasing feature of cities in rich countries[34].

Although the decade of the 1980s was the International Drinking Water Supply and Sanitation Decade, about half the population in urban areas in poor countries, and an even greater proportion in rural areas, still lack safe water and adequate sanitation. The proportion of the world's population provided with safe water and sanitation services increased in the 1980s. During the same period, however, the growth of the population was even greater. In 1991, while about 1.7 billion people in poor countries were served with water through a pipe supply, there still remained one billion people unserved. There were also about 1.7 billion people still without access to appropriate means of sewage disposal[35]. Lack of adequate drinking water particularly affects women. The gender-based division of labour places women more frequently in contact with polluted water and the risk of infection from water-borne diseases.

Water and food pollution in developing countries are caused by poor sanitation, poor hygiene, inadequate waste disposal and water treatment. These conditions create major epidemics of diarrhoeal disease, especially among children. The outbreak of cholera in South America in 1991 was the result of poor sanitary conditions. Global warming may also have contributed by encouraging the growth of surface water algae which protect the cholera bacteria[36]. This cholera outbreak cost Peru about $1 billion, three times the total amount invested in the country's water supply during the previous decade[37].

The World Bank estimates that 80 countries now have water shortages that threaten both health status and national economies. As industrial, agricultural and individual demands escalate, the situation is deteriorating: worldwide the demand for water is doubling every 21 years[37]. The World Bank proposes huge investments in sanitation and water schemes and suggests that water be valued as an economic good, rather than a human right, and water services be privatised. It is unlikely that these suggestions will solve the problems of water supply for the poor; long-term community development projects may be of more benefit.

Malnutrition and deficiency diseases are major problems in poor countries and in some population groups within wealthy countries. The major hazards for both children and adults are protein-energy malnutrition caused by poverty, and vitamin A, iodine and iron deficiencies[38]. Approximately 780 million people (15 % of the total world population) are energy deficient. The worst situation is in Africa which regularly experiences devastating famines with children and women being most at risk. The World Summit for Children goal was for a halving of the 1990 rate of child malnutrition by the year 2000. By mid-decade, it appears that about a half of all poor countries are on target to achieve this goal[8].

Inadequate diet, in association with infectious diseases, accounts for a large share of the world's disease burden, including as much as a quarter of the burden among children. There is also increasing evidence that inadequate nutrition in pregnancy may be an important factor in the development of a range of adult non-communicable disease[39].

The prospect for adequate food supplies to meet the growing world population is not reassuring; distribution of the available food is also a chronic problem. The so called 'green revolution' of the 1970s and 1980s produced optimism, and genetic developments might yet produce further high yield and adaptable crops. Production is now levelling off, however. For example, the growth in rice yields virtually ceased in the Philippines in the latter half of the 1980s[36]. Globally per capita grain production has also fallen[40]. The available land for crop production is limited, the supply of fresh water is dwindling, and the seas have been over fished. The centralisation of large scale agricultural production, often under the control of multi-national businesses, has had an adverse impact on local communities and reduced the viability of small scale farming. It appears likely that widespread malnourishment will increase, especially in sub-Saharan Africa.

Vitamin A (retinol) deficiency is widely prevalent and causes a wide range of childhood health problems, including ulceration of the cornea of the eye and permanent blindness. According to WHO, 13.8 million children have some eye damage because of vitamin A deficiency. Of these, up to half a million go blind each year and two-thirds of the blinded children die[8].

Iron deficiency and iodine deficiency are also widespread with about 460 million and one billion people, respectively, affected. The amount of iron in the diet in poor countries is decreasing rather than increasing. Girls and women are particularly vulnerable. For example, up to 85% of pregnant Indian women are anaemic; even in richer countries about 15% of pregnant women suffer from anaemia. In many societies women face a lifetime of nutritional inequity with severe consequences for the next generation. Severe iodine deficiency causes endemic cretinism, a condition characterised by irreversible mental deficiency. Cretinism affects 5.7 million people and over 20 million suffer lesser degrees of mental retardation caused by iodine deficiency. The estimated impact of iodine deficiency globally is shown in Figure 3.2[8].

A non-governmental organisation was established in 1985 with the aim of eliminating iodine deficiency disorders by the year 2000[41]. The substantial successes of the global partnership created by this initiative indicate the power of selective disease prevention programmes which translate scientific research into international public health action (see Box 3.2). This project demonstrates the application of science to health and development in poor countries. The key factor was that the International Council for the Control of Iodine Deficiency Diseases, a non governmental organisation, was able to successfully advocate with the major international agencies and national governments. It provides one model for translating scientific research to international public health[42].

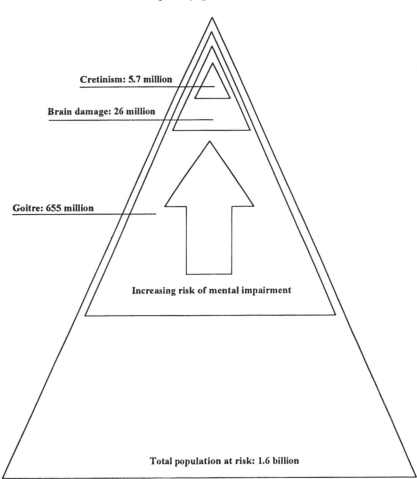

Cretinism: 5.7 million

Brain damage: 26 million

Goitre: 655 million

Increasing risk of mental impairment

Total population at risk: 1.6 billion

The estimated 1.6 billion people at risk represent approximately 30% of the world's population

Figure 3.2. Estimated impact of iodine deficiency worldwide. Source: UNICEF (ref. 8).

3.2.3 Literacy and education

Education is one of the most important and most readily modifiable social determinants of health[19]. Literacy interacts with the availablility of free or inexpensive and effective health services to produce major positive health improvements. Policies to expand schooling are therefore crucial for promoting health, although in the long-term integrated primary health care programmes have the greatest potential. Improvements in the education of girls is increasingly recognised as a central factor in improving maternal and child

---

Box 3.2   Eradicating iodine deficiency disorders: a global partnership[41]

Iodine deficiency is the most common preventable cause of mental deficiency in the world today. WHO estimates that more than one billion are at risk with at least 20 million suffering from mental deficiency which is totally preventable by the correction of iodine deficiency before pregnancy.

Three steps have been identified as crucial for the success of the eradication programme:

1. The establishment of a scientific base and reconceptualisation of the problem as a population concern.
2. Bridging the gap to a public health programme with the creation of a non-governmental organisation made up of the scientific community and public health professionals from a range of disciplines.
3. Development of a global partnership through the United Nations system.

---

health. Unfortunately, levels of literacy and education, especially among women, are still very low in many poor countries. Progress was made in the 1960s and 1970s in increasing the proportion of children completing primary schooling in most poor countries; between 1970 and 1990 the gender gap in education more than halved in poor countries. One of the effects of structural adjustment programmes in the 1980s, however, was that governments were encouraged to reduce educational spending to meet debt repayments[43]. Primary schooling has suffered, particularly in sub-Saharan Africa[8].

Renewed lending by the World Bank for education following the 1993 World Development Report may lead to more progress. The mere provision of loans for education, however, does not inevitably result in increased schooling, especially for girls. Also required is a change in attitude by those in power and a full understanding of the many reasons why parents keep children from school, including the need to supplement the household income. If the position of women in society cannot be changed by modifying religious or cultural practices, it may be changed by encouraging female education and employment[44].

3.3 Global environmental changes

The major new public health hazard is the threat to our long-term existence posed by global damage to the biophysical and ecological environment.

This is the most important new challenge to epidemiology and public health because it transcends national and regional boundaries. The state of the environment is ultimately a much more powerful determinant of health status than either genes or personal behaviour. The underlying problem is the continuing inequality between rich and poor countries. A truly global perspective will be required if public health practitioners are to play a part in the solution to this problem.

Environmental epidemiology has focused attention on the health impact of air pollution, pesticides and toxic chemicals. It has yet to adequately confront the scientific difficulties posed by 'planetary overload'[36] which includes global environmental hazards such as ozone depletion and global warming. The health impact of global environmental change is indirect and not immediately obvious.

In poor countries the immediate health impact of a deteriorating environment is all too apparent: lack of access to safe water, food and sanitation. In wealthy countries the impact is usually more subtle, but ultimately just as important. In many poor urban areas of wealthy countries, the immediate environmental concerns are the same as those facing much of the poor world.

Air pollution is a major health hazard in many major cities of the world[45]. About 1.5 billion people are living in a polluted ambient air environment detrimental to health and this exposure is responsible for about 500 000 excess deaths each year[46]. Air pollution is severe in some areas of Central and Eastern Europe, although only limited data are available to estimate its health impact. It is possible that in the Czech Republic, one of the most heavily polluted countries, air pollution may be responsible for up to 3% of all deaths; this is less than 10% of the mortality gap between this country and Western Europe[47]. Large cities in poor countries are usually the worst off, with pollution levels similar to those of the severely polluted cities of the wealthy countries about 40 years ago. Air pollution is increasing in many urban areas and an increase in mortality and morbidity, especially from chronic respiratory diseases, is likely.

The health hazards of industrial and agricultural chemicals and the toxic waste created by their production and use, also pose increasing problems. Episodes of poisoning because of industrial errors have been catastrophic. For example, in Bhopal, India, at least 3500 people died and 200 000 were injured in 1984 when isocyonate was released from a pesticide factory into the surrounding slums. The impact of this disaster continues to be felt, although there is no accurate record of the number of people whose health has been permanently impaired[48]. Attempts to adequately compensate the victims of this disaster have not yet been successful[49]. It is likely that, as poor countries continue to industrialise and embrace consumerism and western notions of development, there will be more Bhopal-like disasters[4]. A particularly worrying concern is the increasing number of nuclear reactors which have the potential to expose large numbers of people to ionising radiation (see Box 3.3).

Box 3.3   Health consequences of the Chernobyl accident[5]

- The largest ever radiation accident involving a nuclear reactor occurred on 26 April 1986 at the Chernobyl nuclear power plant in the Ukraine; five million people in the Ukraine, Belarus and the Russian Federation were exposed to ionising radiation.
- At the time of the accident, 300 of the 444 people at the reactor site were admitted to hospital, 134 of whom were diagnosed as having acute radiation sickness; 28 of these died within three months and one-third of the remainder suffered various disorders.
- Psychological effects, believed to be unrelated to direct radiation exposure, resulted from the lack of information immediately after the accident, the stress and trauma of compulsory relocation to less contaminated areas, the break in social ties, and the fear that radiation exposure could cause health damage in the future.
- An increase in the incidence of childhood thyroid cancer has been one of the major health consequences of the accident, particularly in Belarus.
- Ultimately it is estimated that the after effects of this nuclear disaster will cause 6,600 more deaths from cancer and leukaemia.

The newest and most threatening environmental hazards are global warming and the depletion of the stratospheric ozone layer by pollution and the release of chemicals, particularly chlorofluorocarbons used in refrigeration fluids, into the environment. Ironically, it was the accumulation of stratospheric ozone that shielded the earth from damaging ultraviolet light and thus enabled the evolution of species[36]. Most of the ozone-destroying chemicals and greenhouse gases come from wealthy countries.

Ozone layer depletion will lead to greater exposure to incoming solar ultraviolet radiation. The direct health effects of ozone depletion include an increase in the risk of skin cancer and cataract. Greater indirect effects, however, could result through damage to the food chain.

The 'greenhouse' effect or global warming is caused by carbon dioxide and other gases that trap heat radiation from the earth's surface and lead to global warming. The effects of global warming are more long-term, more damaging, and more difficult to prevent than ozone depletion. The health impact of climatic and other environmental changes includes an increase in the global population exposed to vector-borne diseases[51]. Global warming may also raise ocean levels and have a variety of effects on crop production[52]. In addition, there are already at least 25 million people who can no longer gain a secure livelihood in their homelands because of drought, soil erosion, desertification, deforestation and other environmental problems. These environmental refugees will increase dramatically unless the motivation to migrate is reduced by supplying them with acceptable lifestyles[53].

These global environmental changes have generated much debate, including at the 1992 Earth Summit which produced Agenda 21, an environmental agenda for the next century (see Box 3.4). In part, this debate is a result of inadequate and often conflicting information.

Box 3.4   Agenda 21: a strategy for change[10]

Areas in which international commitment to change is needed:

- allocating international aid to programs directed at poverty alleviation and environmental health;
- investing in efforts to reduce soil erosion and to put agricultural practices on a sustainable footing;
- allocating more resources for family planning and education, especially for girls;
- supporting governments in their attempts to remove distortions and macroeconomic imbalances that damage the environment;
- providing finance to protect natural habitat and biodiversity;
- investing in research and development of non-carbon energy alternatives to respond to climate change.

Calls for action have come mainly from wealthy countries, although the environmental effects will ultimately be experienced globally. Epidemiological data are sparse in this area. Interdisciplinary collaboration and methods for estimating long-term effects on the basis of theoretical models require development. Predictions made over the last few years on the basis of global warming have been accurate. In 1995, the Inter-governmental Panel on Climate Change confirmed that the warming of the past few years 'is unlikely to be entirely due to natural causes' and that 'a pattern of climate response to human activities is identifiable in the climatological record'[55].

The solution to these global environmental changes includes population control and reducing dependence on cheap fossil fuels as a source of energy. Of more fundamental importance is sustainable development and the redistribution of global wealth to prevent the further destruction of the environment, especially in poor countries. The global response has, however, been low key and preventive actions on a scale to conserve the environment have not yet matched the rhetoric, apart from a few exceptions. In 1987, 36 nations signed the Montreal Protocol and agreed to restrict their release (but not production) of ozone damaging chemicals with the aim of halving the release of chlorofluorocarbons by the year 2000. This Protocol was noteworthy because the evidence linking ozone depletion to adverse health effects was theoretical, and the empirical evidence non-existent; the decision was taken even before the ozone damaging effect of these chemicals was confirmed. The Montreal Protocol was revised and strengthened in 1990 and again in 1992. A halving of the peak 1988 emission levels of chlorofluorocarbons has been achieved in a few years as a result of this concerted global effort[36]. This positive development indicates that, where political will is strong, progress is possible. The Montreal Protocol is now faced with its first cases of defaulters and evasion of the controls is occurring with the rapid growth of the black market[56].

3.4 Population growth and over consumption

3.4.1 Population growth

Underlying the adverse global environmental changes are two fundamental issues: rapidly increasing population in poor countries and over consumption in rich countries. The exponential population growth of the last ten generations will lead to either a levelling off because of actions taken now, or a dramatic reduction because of environmental disaster, if no action is taken. Population growth is indisputably a public health issue[57]. Public health programmes are a central means for stabilising or reducing population growth.

Globally, world population growth is slowing from an annual rate of increase of 2.1% in the late 1960s to about 1.7% in the 1990s reflecting the substantial decline in total fertility rate (Table 3.2)[7]. Growth rates are expected to continue their decline to reach an average annual rate of population increase of about 1% by about the year 2020. Population growth is

Table 3.2 *Reductions in total fertility rate (live births per woman), 1970–92*[7]

Country	1970	1992
Wealthy countries	2.3	1.9
Poor countries	5.7	3.5
Sub-Saharan Africa	6.6	6.3
Middle Eastern Countries	6.8	4.8
East Asia	5.3	1.9
SE Asia and Pacific	5.6	3.3
South Asia	5.9	4.1
Latin America/Caribbean	5.3	3.1

still considerably higher in the poor world (2.1% per year between 1985 and 1990) compared with the wealthy countries (0.6% per year). In the poorest countries the average rate of population growth increased, and over the last five years averaged 2.8% per year[58].

The world's population is growing at a rate of almost 100 million a year with 90% occurring in poor countries[59]. The Indian population contributes almost one in five of the world's total increase in population each year. A new policy to control population growth proposed by an expert group in India is said to be 'pro-nature, pro-poor and pro-women'[60]. The policy aims to replace vertically structured and target-oriented family planning welfare systems with people-oriented, decentralised and democratic planning involving village and city councils as well as state legislatures. Not all aspects of the proposed policy have been supported by members of women's organisations who have been the recipients of coercive programmes in the past.

Several countries in sub-Saharan Africa may already have entered the demographic trap where rapid population growth, as a result of falling death rates and sustained high birth rates, results in increasing pressure on resources, a rapidly deteriorating environment and ultimately an increase in infant death rates[61]. This has been called 'entrapment'[62] (Box 3.5). One essential requirement for preventing this process is a radical reduction of fertility. The alternative, external reliance on provision of food, can, at best, be only a short-term solution and runs the risk of encouraging starvation or warfare, as is the case in Rwanda[63].

A critical feature is the ultimate size of a population at the end of its demographic transition in relation to its carrying capacity and its connectedness. The central importance of child survival instead of family planning and development, poses important ethical questions which have not yet been adequately addressed at an international level[64–66]. For example, while UNICEF

Box 3.5   Demographic entrapment[62]

'A local population is demographically trapped if it has exceeded, or is projected to exceed, the combination of:

- *the carrying capacity of its own ecosystem;*
- *its ability to obtain the products, and particularly the food, produced by other ecosystems except as food aid;*
- *its ability to migrate to other ecosystems in a manner which preserves (or improves) its standard of living.*

The first two conditions describe the links that a population has with other ecosystems, and are crucial. They are most easily thought of as 'connectedness', and its opposite 'disconnectedness'. A severely trapped population faces the four tragedies of entrapment in varying combinations. Depending on local cultural, political and ecological factors it can starve, die from disease, slaughter itself or its neighbours, or be supported indefinitely by food aid'.

---

has emphasised the close interaction between poverty, population growth and environmental degradation[8], it disputes the poverty trap and is reluctant to recognise that aid directed towards reducing child death rates may be aggravating the effects of population growth, especially in the absence of fertility reduction which requires substantial social and economic resources[62].

China provides an example of what has been done in one poor country to avoid entrapment. Population growth has been limited with the official one child per family policy established in 1979. There are a number of unexpected outcomes of this policy in the short term, and in the long term it means that China will age sooner and more quickly than most other poor countries.

There is controversy on the nature of the relationship between poverty and population growth. Some biologists suggest the central problem is high birth rates. Others suggest that poverty is the force behind high birth rates, either because parents need more children for their own (economic) survival in later life, or because of a real sense of despair and lack of control. These two competing explanations have profoundly different policy implications. From a practical point of view, evidence favours the importance of making contraception available because there is general agreement that rapid population growth impedes social and economic progress[67]. Ultimately, of course, the solution must lie in the integration of both approaches – more equitable distribution of wealth and the provision of reproductive health care (Box 3.6).

Box 3.6　The reproductive revolution

Bangladesh is a good example of the so called 'reproductive revolution'[68]. Despite being one of the world's poorest nations with high child mortality, and a society where most families depend on children for labour and support in old age, fertility rates declined from 7 to 5.5 children per woman between 1970 and 1990. During the same period, the use of contraception increased from 3 to 40%. Bangladesh has a high literacy rate (78%) and basic literacy and women's education are important factors in increasing the use of contraceptives. The availability of contraceptives in the context of quality integrated health care and real freedom of choice are essential.

In many parts of the world religion and politics have all too often taken precedence over public health concerns. Women in much of Central and Eastern Europe, particularly in Romania, have relied heavily on unsafe abortion because of the enforced scarcity of suitable contraception and safe abortion services. In the United States of America and elsewhere, women's legal right to safe abortion services is constantly under threat.

At present, only about 1% of all foreign aid is devoted to international family planning. Double this amount would be sufficient to make contraceptive choices universally available before the end of century. About 100 million couples around the world want to limit the size of their families but cannot gain access to family planning services[69]. Cultural and religious beliefs hinder progress in this area. In 1996 the budget for the US Agency for International Development, a long-term leader in international family planning, was cut by almost seven-eighths; this cut will have major adverse effects on the health of women and families worldwide[70].

As we have seen in Chapter 2, diseases and deaths related to pregnancy complications cause substantial preventable mortality and morbidity. Births to very young women, closely spaced births and frequent pregnancies, inadequate prenatal and natal care, unwanted pregnancies that lead to unsafe and often illegal abortion, and malnutrition, all increase the risks of pregnancy. Women in some poor countries spend over half their childbearing years either pregnant or breast feeding[71]. For most of these women reproductive health is inseparable from general health. Maternal mortality is clearly responsive to social and political changes as the Romanian experience, described in Chapter 2, dramatically demonstrates.

In mid-1994 the world's population was 5.7 billion people. The highest projection by the United Nations Population Fund suggests that by the year 2050, there will be a staggering 12.5 billion. At the 1994 United Nations Conference in Cairo on Population and Development, guidelines were adopted to contain the world's population at about 7.3 billion by the year 2015, and 7.8 billion in the year 2050. The Conference polarised secular liberals and religious conservatives who had serious reservations about references to abortion, the family, and sex education in the 20 year draft programme of action. Fortunately, a positive compromise was reached and a programme of action endorsed. The programme is farsighted and, apart from birth control, acknowledges the importance of the status of women, education, sexually transmitted diseases, health care, population distribution, and migration[67]. The recommendations of the conference are, of course, non-binding, and the impact on population growth, as well as the more general targets, may be limited.

3.4.2 *Over consumption*

Over consumption of energy, the other fundamental cause of global environmental degradation, is a defining feature of the rich world[72], and is growing at a faster rate than the population. As energy consumption increases as populations grow and as poor people become richer, economic growth has the potential of hugely increasing energy consumption in poor countries, even with only a modest rise in the standard of living. This rise in energy consumption and the associated rise in carbon dioxide concentrations will contribute further to global warming. A narrow focus on economic growth is shortsighted.

Both the rich and the poor worlds have a role to play. The rich world needs to limit its carbon dioxide production and share its food and other resources. The poor world needs to limit its population. Both rich and poor have to adopt a sustainable life-style[61,73]. Logically, however, given that 20% of the world's population consumes 80% of the resources, the initiatives must come from the rich world. Unfortunately, the prospects for this leadership are slim: it may take a global crisis of huge proportions for wealthy countries to take seriously their responsibility for the future of the world's poor.

3.5 Personal behaviours and health

The focus of epidemiological research over the last five decades has been on the association of personal behaviours with non-communicable disease.

Table 3.3 *Distribution of adult smokers in wealthy and poor countries, 1995*[74]

	Men		Women		Total	
	Millions	%	Millions	%	Millions	%
Wealthy countries	200	41	100	21	300	30
Poor countries	700	50	100	8	800	35
Total	900	48	200	12	1100	33

This research has been enormously productive, although it has too often led to preventive programmes which blame individuals for their unhealthy habits (or lifestyles), rather than the powerful social and economic forces which condition these behaviours. Research on the role of individual human behaviours has undoubtedly been of great value in identifying specific risk factors. This information has been of primary benefit to privileged groups within wealthy countries. A focus on individual risk factors identifies only one of the pathways to disease. A major challenge is the integration of epidemiological research with research from other disciplines to clarify the other important influences on pathways to health (see Chapter 6).

3.5.1 *Tobacco smoking*

The products of the tobacco industry are the most readily preventable modern cause of premature death and disease. Tobacco has been used for centuries, although it was not until the development of mass production and marketing techniques that the habit became widespread. There are more than one billion smokers in the world today, the majority of whom live in poor countries (Table 3.3)[74].

The per capita consumption of tobacco peaked in some countries of Western Europe, North America and Australasia over three decades ago and has been declining in many of these countries, although the decline may have stopped in the 1990s[75]. A feature of the tobacco market in wealthy countries is the growth in the consumption by young people, especially women, even where consumption is declining in men and older people[76]. Lung cancer has already overtaken breast cancer as the leading cause of cancer death in women in the United States of America, and the worldwide lung cancer epidemic is still evolving.

Another important aspect of smoking trends in wealthy countries is the widening social class gradients in cigarette smoking. Although smoking used to be a habit of wealthy people, this has not been the case over the last few decades. Since the first authoritative public health campaigns of the early 1960s, privileged groups have increasingly given up smoking and overall smoking prevalence has declined. This widening inequality by social class gradients is one example of the unintended effects of a health policy which does not consider the complexity of the social circumstances in which individuals make personal health choices.

The epidemiological data on smoking points to a more general paradox: people whose health is already at risk through the cumulative effects of social and economic disadvantage are the most likely to pursue unhealthy patterns of behaviour[77]. This is paradoxical only if health behaviours are considered in individualistic terms without considering the social context; nor is this approach helpful in understanding why people, often women, pursue lifestyles that damage their health. Women and poor people generally develop routines that reflect a daily struggle to meet a set of conflicting health needs which are related to the welfare of an entire household. Health choices reflect a compromise which maintains household routines[77]. In this context, smoking by young and disadvantaged women is one means by which the welfare of the family is promoted, despite its long-term adverse health effects on the individual. Among many low income families, smoking is one of the few luxuries and remains the norm[78].

Of great concern is the steady rise in consumption in poor countries stimulated by the profit-seeking multi-national tobacco industry. The poor world is particularly vulnerable to the tactics of the tobacco industry. In many poor countries tobacco is considered an 'affordable luxury' for people with few educational or employment opportunities. In a Chinese survey more than two-thirds of men were smokers (but only 2% of women) and smokers spent a substantial proportion of their income on cigarettes; there was a low rate of quitting and a low desire to quit[79]. Reprehensibly, the government of the United States of America has used the threat of trade sanctions to open up domestic cigarette markets in many countries to multi-national tobacco companies. In many countries tobacco is an important cash crop and a source of export earnings; tobacco is the most widely grown non-food crop in many African countries[80]. Zimbabwe, for example, is the second largest exporter of tobacco leaf in the world and derives more than a quarter of its export earnings from the crop[81]. Tobacco tax revenue is attractive to all governments, especially those of impoverished and indebted countries.

Tobacco production is directly responsible for other important adverse consequences apart from health effects. For most countries, tobacco is responsible for a deficit in the balance of trade. Some of the poorest nations use precious capital to purchase tobacco and deforestation is a serious and rapidly growing problem.

Tobacco advertising is widespread and subject to few controls. There is evidence from at least one poor county, Papua New Guinea, that a systematic price policy not only reduces consumption but also increases national tax receipts for many years before a point of diminishing return is reached[82]. This relationship is well described for rich countries, although the point of diminishing returns to government revenue may soon be reached. There is conflicting evidence as to whether an increase in the price of cigarettes only makes poor families poorer or encourages them to stop smoking[78,83]. The long-term solution is to deal with the underlying poverty and the lack of esteem amongst poor families. In the short term, the development and the evaluation of smoking cessation programmes of relevance to disadvantaged people is a priority..

The adverse health consequences of tobacco have been endlessly documented over the last 50 years by epidemiologists. This evidence is accepted by all but the tobacco industry and its special consultants. The impact of tobacco on health is staggering. Worldwide, about three million adults die each year from tobacco-caused diseases. About ten million people (mostly in China and India) will die each year by the year 2025. It is salutary to note that these ten million people are now alive (and smoking) and could be prevented from dying prematurely. The epidemic of smoking-caused deaths in women has not yet reached its peak anywhere. Death from smoking has become common in women in only a few countries. The proportion of women eventually killed by tobacco will be similar to that in men if they continue to smoke, as has happened in Denmark (Figure 3.3)[84].

The decline in consumption in wealthy countries is a result of public health campaigns and comprehensive tobacco control policies which have evolved through the efforts of coalitions of special interest groups and the support of some governments. Most efforts, however, have been directed towards the regulation of the behaviour of individuals, rather than control of the tobacco industry. The 1994 World Conference on Tobacco and Health held in Paris encouraged all nations to implement the comprehensive international strategies for tobacco control. A regional example is shown in Box 3.7.

Litigation, at least in wealthy countries, may have a major impact on future consumption trends. To date, tobacco companies have been successful in winning law suits claiming damages for smoking-caused illnesses, although the tide has turned as the emphasis shifts from individual law suits

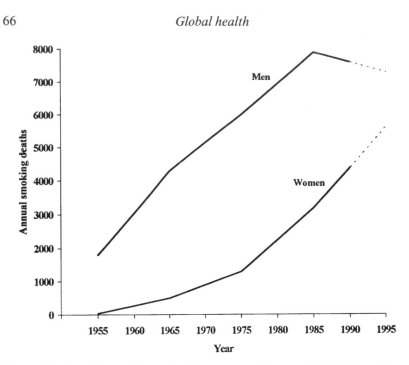

Figure 3.3. Smoking-attributed deaths per year in Denmark, 1955–95. Estimated (. . .). Source: Peto R, *et al.* (ref. 84).

Box 3.7 Action plan on Tobacco or Health for 1995–99

The action plan on Tobacco or Health for the Western Pacific region of the WHO calls for all governments to implement comprehensive tobacco control measures by 1999[85,86]. These include:

• a national policy and central co-ordinating agency on tobacco or health;
• health education;
• comprehensive tobacco control legislation; and
• pricing policy.

Specific goals for countries and areas with a long history of tobacco or health action is to decrease tobacco consumption by at least 1–2% per year and for other countries to implement national action plans to reduce smoking.

to class action suits. For example, five US states have recovered from a small cigarette manufacturer millions of dollars spent on the treatment of cigarette-caused diseases[87,88]. A positive side-effect of this litigation will be the need for tobacco companies to increase the price of cigarettes and this in turn will deter young smokers; a possible negative effect would be an increasing dependence of state governments on tobacco revenue.

In summary, despite the enormous success of epidemiology in identifying the extent of the tobacco induced epidemics, from a global perspective prevention policies have had only limited success. The lesson from wealthy countries is that changing addictive behaviour requires intensive effort to build a social movement at a non-governmental level which, when strong, will lead to government policy changes[89]. Public health practitioners have so far failed to deal with this most preventable cause of premature death and disease largely because of the focus on individual behaviours and their associated risks rather than on the economic, social and cultural determinants of the tobacco epidemics.

3.5.2 Alcohol

The consumption of alcohol, especially by men, is widespread in most societies. The adverse health effects of alcohol consumption are many and varied, although in contrast to tobacco there are some beneficial effects. In most countries, important health problems stem from the excessive consumption of alcohol by a small proportion of the population. In New Zealand, for example, 11% of the population drinks over half the total alcohol consumed, and young men make up most of this high risk group[90]. Excessive consumption is dangerous. Combined with other activities such as driving, it becomes even more dangerous, both to the drinker and to others. Although alcohol related problems are more frequent in heavy drinkers, the moderate drinking segment of the population, a much larger group, contributes the greater proportion of the problems. Effective strategies for the prevention and control of alcohol induced health and social problems must focus on all drinkers, not just the small segment of the population at most risk[91].

Alcohol related diseases affect 5 to 10% of the world's population and was estimated to account for about 3% of the global burden of disease in 1990[6], although this is probably an underestimate. There is still much to be learnt about the balance between the adverse and beneficial social and health consequences of alcohol consumption. The protective effects against coronary heart disease, for example, appear real but are only of public health importance in older people who are at an increased risk of cardio-vascular disease[92]. In some countries alcohol is responsible for about 20% of all deaths among 15–34 year old people; in older age groups there is a possible beneficial impact of moderate alcohol intake on reducing coronary heart disease death rates[90]. On balance, it is likely that alcohol is respons-ible for about 500000 excess deaths worldwide, most from injury; the adverse disease effects are equal to the preventive effects on cardiovascular disease[93].

Average alcohol consumption increased between 1950 and 1980, partic-ularly in poor countries which started from low levels of consumption. Since then, per capita consumption has levelled off, especially in wealthy countries. A particularly worrying feature of the alcohol scene is the young age at which many people begin drinking. Heavy consumption by young people is, to a large extent, a response to social ostracism and the despair resulting from unemployment and the lack of prospects.

The alcohol industry is powerful and pervasive. Alcohol advertising has firmly established the industry as an important and accepted sponsor of many sporting events. It is not surprising that attempts to control alcohol advertising have met with little success. The alcohol industry remains the main barrier to the prevention of alcohol related mortality and morbidity. A range of strategies are available to prevent alcohol problems. Strong com-munity and government leadership is required to implement these policies.

3.5.3 Dietary imbalance: underconsumption and overconsumption

Malnutrition resulting from lack of food is the major dietary problem worldwide and is responsible for a significant part of the global burden of disease[6]. As countries become richer, however, consumption of animal fat replaces traditional foods which are generally of lower fat and higher car-bohydrate content. The relationship between diet and non-communicable disease is complex, but the increased consumption of fat is the major under-lying cause of the modern epidemic of coronary heart disease. Vegetarians have lower mortality largely because of their low intake of animal fat. More generally, the affluent high meat eating quarter of the world's population is not ecologically desirable at a global level, because of the large amount of edible energy required to produce animal products[94].

Increased salt intake, along with excessive body weight and alcohol intake, is responsible for the high average levels of blood pressure in wealthy countries. An imbalance between intake of calories and levels of activity, results in the increasing prevalence of obesity observed in many countries. In some countries, average energy intake has declined as obesity rates have increased suggesting that levels of physical activity have declined even faster[95]. Obesity has a variety of adverse health effects including raised blood pressure, diabetes, heart disease, and joint problems. A range of other dietary components are implicated in a variety of modern diseases, for example calcium intake and osteoporosis, but collectively they are of much less public health significance than the major non-communicable diseases such as heart disease, stroke and cancer. Public health practitioners in wealthy countries are rightly concerned about the health effects of over-nutrition, but it must be remembered that from a global perspective, hunger is much more important.

3.5.4 Physical inactivity

The increasing prevalence of physical inactivity in wealthy countries illustrates the manner in which economic development adversely influences health. Traditionally most people were physically active. In some societies this pattern is still widespread. Physical activity, however, has become a leisure time activity undertaken in wealthy countries by only a small (and usually the most advantaged) proportion of the population. In the United States of America, for example, only about 20% of adults undertake regular physical activity sufficient to confer health benefits[96].

Overall, physical inactivity is responsible for about 2% of the global burden of disease[93]. The epidemiological evidence on the adverse effects of physical inactivity is now persuasive. Physical inactivity is strongly associated with increased risks of various conditions including heart disease, stroke, some cancers, diabetes and osteoporosis. The relationship between inactivity and heart disease is probably causal. Inactivity is so common that it is likely to be responsible for approximately 30% of new cases of heart disease in many countries[97]. Although the benefits of physical activity increase with the amount and duration of activity, relatively small amounts (for example, up to 20 minutes three times a week) are worthwhile. Incorporating even this small amount of activity into daily life in wealthy countries is surprisingly difficult and not made easier by dependence on personalised transport. Guidelines addressed to the population as a whole now emphasise the importance of encouraging sedentary people to walk on a regular basis, rather than the less feasible goal of more vigorous activity[96].

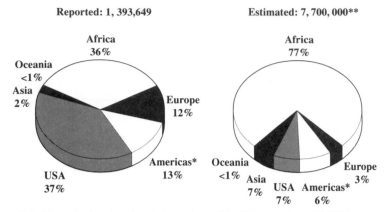

Figure 3.4. Reported and estimated number of AIDS cases by mid 1996.
*Excluding United States of America; **Adjusted following review of global
estimates. Source: WHO (ref. 98).

3.5.5 Unsafe sex

Sexually transmitted diseases have always been prevalent. The advent of the
human immunodeficiency virus (HIV), responsible for AIDS, however,
added a new and cruel dimension to sexual activity. HIV/AIDS indicates
our vulnerability to emerging microbes. HIV infection is spread in a variety
of ways, but the major modes are via sexual intercourse and intravenous
drug use. The major risk factors for HIV are unsafe injecting habits, multiple sexual partners, and unsafe sexual practices, especially intercourse
without the use of condoms or other barrier methods of protection.

Approximately 80% of HIV infected people develop AIDS within 15
years. Only a very small proportion of HIV infected people (3–7%) do not
progress to AIDS. There is no effective cure or preventive immunisation.
Most AIDS patients die; the case fatality five years from diagnosis is
approximately 95%.

The first case of AIDS was diagnosed in 1981. The AIDS epidemic began
at a time when wealthy countries were becoming complacent about infectious diseases. Not since the 1918 influenza pandemic had such a devastating epidemic appeared. By mid 1996, almost eight million cases of AIDS
had occurred, two million in 1995 alone, and about 17 million adults and
1.5 million children had been infected with HIV (Figure 3.4)[98]. There is a
large discrepancy between the reported and estimated number of AIDS
cases because of under diagnosis, incomplete reporting, and reporting
delay. The number of HIV infected people is expected to rise to about 40
million by the year 2000, and the total death toll from AIDS is expected to
exceed eight million by the year 2000.

The public health impact of the AIDS epidemic is chilling. For example, by the year 2010, it is expected that AIDS will have lowered the life expectancy in Zambia to 33 years from 66 years, and to 40 years from 70 years in Zimbabwe[99]. The world had little readiness, either politically or socially, to confront the public health crises which rapidly developed in the 1980s as the epidemic spread. The epidemic was initially categorised as a disease specific to homosexual men who suffered stigmatisation and additional discrimination. It took time to reduce the prejudice and bureaucratic inertia that characterised the initial response of most governments. It is especially tragic that the lessons learnt in the United States of America and Europe have been so slowly applied in other regions.

The rate of development of new AIDS cases has largely levelled off in Europe, the United States of America and other western countries, possibly because of changing behaviour and secure blood supplies. The virus continues to ravage sub-Saharan Africa, however, and is rapidly spreading through Asia[98]. In some countries of sub-Saharan Africa, AIDS is the commonest cause of death in young men and women and this is now also the case in parts of the United States of America. In many poor countries, up to two-thirds of all new HIV infections are occurring in people aged 15–24 years; a third of the new cases in 1993 occurred in Asia. A particular cause of concern now is China, with its huge population undergoing rapid social change and with HIV already making inroads in the southern provinces[100]. Similarly, an expanding HIV epidemic continues in India. The consequences could be catastrophic; by the year 2000 it is predicted that one million people will have AIDS in India and another five million will be HIV positive[101].

Epidemiology has played a prime role in identifying HIV and tracking the spread of the AIDS pandemic. There are three broad epidemiological patterns to this epidemic[102]. In the United States of America, Canada, Western Europe, Australia, North Africa and parts of South America, HIV has spread mainly among homosexual and bisexual men and injecting drug users. In the remainder of Africa and in South America, where multiple sexual partners are common, most infections have been acquired heterosexually. The third pattern is found in the Asian-Pacific, Eastern European, and the Middle Eastern areas where HIV was introduced later.

Social and demographic factors greatly affect the spread of HIV. In many poor countries male migration to more wealthy countries in search of work is common and economically impoverished women are forced to move to urban areas and become sex workers to earn money for their poor rural families. The task of convincing apparently healthy young men and women to practice safe sex by using condoms and barrier methods is difficult, especially given the lack of availability and unacceptability of family planning in many parts of the world.

An important change in the international campaign against AIDS was the replacement of WHO's Global AIDS programme in 1995 by a new structure (UNAIDS) representing all United Nations agencies dealing with the epidemic[103]. The purpose of the change is to avoid conflicts of interest and duplication of efforts. Of equal importance is the recognition that the AIDS epidemic is now at a critical juncture. In many countries, boredom with AIDS is setting in and resources are not adequate for the sustained prevention and education programmes that are required. In some countries the focus is shifting to the heterosexual epidemic and prevention among homosexual and bisexual men is being neglected. Few communities have achieved a level of behaviour change sufficient to halt the spread of HIV. The demonstration that treatment of other sexually transmitted diseases with relatively cheap interventions also slows the transmission of HIV, offers some hope for the future[104].

An important insight from over a decade of prevention and control efforts is the critical relationship between social discrimination and vulnerability to HIV. This discrimination interferes with every aspect of prevention and control programmes. The Global AIDS Policy Coalition has prepared a new strategy to reduce the widening gap between the pandemic and the response[105,106]. This strategy is based on the recognition that social forces shape personal and collective vulnerability to HIV/AIDS and provides an excellent outline of an appropriate response to a global problem.

3.6 Injury: unintentional and intentional

Injuries are a major and increasing cause of death and disability in all countries. Although individuals are often blamed for their injuries, in most cases there are powerful environmental forces responsible for the incident leading to the injury.

3.6.1 Car crashes

In many rich countries, cars are an indispensable aspect of daily life for much of the population. These societies are organised on the assumption that personal transport is readily available. The widespread use of motor cars is a mixed blessing. Car crashes are an important cause of death, responsible for about one million deaths worldwide each year[6]. The numbers killed in car crashes is not high in comparison, say, with heart disease, but the people killed are usually young. As the number of cars increases, so too does the number of deaths; on average one person is killed each year for every 400 vehicles[107].

The type of injury varies according to the type of vehicle most commonly used. In countries with a high proportion of motorcycles, for example Southeast Asia, the risks are greater for drivers or passengers, but lower for pedestrians. In wealthy countries the highest crash death rate is among young men, reflecting car ownership patterns and high risk behaviours such as drinking and driving.

Future trends in motor vehicle crash death rates in poor countries will depend on traffic densities and on the initiation and effectiveness of preventive measures. In many rich countries death rates are declining, despite increasing traffic densities, because of the gradual introduction of safety measures and the general economic slowdown which reduces road travel. Public health campaigns and legislation, for example prelicence training, drink-driving laws including random breath tests, control of speeding, compulsory wearing of seat belts, vehicle design requirements, road improvements and better management of injuries, have all been effective. Thus, although there is an increasing exposure to motor vehicles, the risk of death can be reduced, even if at great cost. It remains to be seen whether the same methods will control the expected increase in road death rates in poor countries as motorised transport becomes increasingly available.

3.6.2 Occupational hazards

Occupational deaths and injuries are more common in poor countries where workers do not have the benefit of occupational health and safety standards. Worldwide, at least 68 million cases of occupational disease injuries occur each year, 145000 of which are fatal[109]. These figures are likely to be serious underestimates because of the limited data from most countries. In total, occupational injuries are responsible for about 3% of the global burden of disease[6].

Injuries are common in occupations associated with agriculture, transportation, construction, and primary industries such as mining[109]. In wealthy countries, the dangers of mining and the high cost of accidents to productivity have been recognised, and this, together with strong unions, has made mining relatively safe. Some of the most spectacular occupational disasters in recent years have resulted from fires in crowded unsafe factories in poor countries, events which ceased to be common in wealthy countries in the early years of this century. New occupational disorders, such as occupational overuse syndrome (or repetitive strain injury), continue to emerge and reflect the changing patterns of employment. In poor countries the rapidity of industrialisation permitted little time for adjustment and workforce training, resulting in considerably higher rates of industrial injuries and occupational diseases than in wealthy countries. The problem is exacerbated by the selective transfer of hazardous industries and chemicals to poor countries, often in the absence of adequate safety measures[4].

3.6.3 *Violence: personal, civil and international*

Violent death is an all too common feature of daily life. Violence takes many forms, and may be self-directed (suicide), family-directed (child or spouse abuse and murder), random (drive-by killings), or directed at ethnic, cultural or national enemies. Suicide is an important cause of death, especially among young men; the causes are complex and the preventive remedies elusive. In many countries suicide rates are increasing. Homicide in many societies usually involves family members, although the pattern varies. In general, rates are highest in young men, especially black men in the United States of America, but rates vary by income, residence and ethnicity and relate closely to the availability of firearms[110]. Gunfire is the second leading cause of death among people aged 4–19 years in the United States of America[111]. Violence against women is pervasive in all societies (see Box 3.8).

The impact of war on health has a depressingly long history. Even more appalling is the continuing resort to warfare to solve territorial, ethnic or cultural conflict. The recent experience in the territories of the former Yugoslavia in the heart of Europe is particularly tragic and does not auger well for peaceful conflict resolution elsewhere. A public health assessment in Bosnia-Herzegovenia revealed extreme disruption to basic health services, mass displacement, severe food shortages, and widespread destruction of public water and sanitation systems[113]. War related violence was the most important public health risk; civilians on all sides of the conflict have been intentional targets of physical and sexual violence. Apart from this direct effect, the war had an indirect impact on health with a doubling of child mortality rates in some areas over a two year period. Between 1945 and 1992, there were 149 major wars, killing more than 23 million people; on an average yearly basis, the number of war deaths in this period was more than double the deaths in the nineteenth century, and seven times greater than in the eighteenth century[114].

War is now mainly an intrastate affair. Of the 82 major armed conflicts

---

Box 3.8 Violence against women: a violation of human rights

Violence against women is a pervasive but little recognised human rights abuse. It ranges from wife or partner abuse to mutilation of girls' genitals to ensure virginity until marriage, to murder of young brides when parents fail to provide expected dowries. The key feature in all of these cases is that women are targets for violence simply because they are female.

Assaults on women by their husbands or male partners are the most common form of violence. It is estimated that about a quarter of the world's women are abused within their own homes. The health consequences of violence include not just physical injury, but psychiatric disturbance and major depression often leading to attempted suicide. Pregnant mothers are prime targets for abuse and women battered during pregnancy have a twofold risk of miscarriage and a fourfold risk of having a low birthweight baby compared with women who are not beaten[112].

Violence (or the threat of violence) is all too common a dimension of sexual decision making, including the use of family planning. The international initiative on safe pregnancy and childbirth, Safe Motherhood, could well extend its brief to include the physical safety of the mother and her child. Similarly, UNICEF and other agencies involved with child survival initiatives could place family violence higher on the international agenda. Ultimately, this would place value on the quality of women's lives.

---

which took place between 1989 and 1992, all but three occurred within states. These conflicts have left more than 40 million people either refugees or displaced in their own countries – double the number a decade ago[7]. Between 1982 and 1992, warfare claimed the lives of 1.5 million children and left another 4.5 million disabled[8].

In mid-1996 there were at least 30 ongoing wars. Modern war is waged primarily against non-combatants; most of those killed or injured are civilians, not directly involved in the fighting. The proliferation of antipersonnel mines means that the after effects of active warfare continue for years[115,116]. The traditional tools of public health are powerless to reduce the impact of war on the population; the international public health communities urgently need to explore methods for promoting sustainable peace.

3.7 Summary

The most important causes of ill health in all countries are the underlying
social and economic characteristics of a society. Unfortunately, these
factors are poorly defined and, from a policy perspective, too often
neglected. A basic and surprisingly low level of wealth is an essential
requirement for health; income distribution within a country seems to be
an important determinant of overall health status. Environmental degradation, caused by over population and over consumption, presents a special
challenge for epidemiology and public health.

The pathways between the social and economic characteristics of a
society and health and disease status are complex and require further multi-
disciplinary study. Much more attention has been directed towards the role
of individual health behaviours. The most readily preventable of these is
tobacco smoking: unfortunately the tobacco epidemic is rapidly spreading
in poor countries. Although much is known about the general and specific
causes of health and disease, this information is insufficiently integrated
into public health policy and practice. As a consequence, the burden of preventable death and disease remains high in all countries.

Chapter 3   Key Points

- The major global public health problem is poverty. The absolute number
  of people living in poverty is increasing.
- Other important socioeconomic determinants of health status are: poor
  housing; unsafe water supply; lack of sanitation; malnutrition; and
  illiteracy.
- The major new public health hazards are the global environmental
  changes: global warming and ozone depletion.
- Rapid population growth, especially in poor countries, and
  overconsumption in wealthy countries, are interrelated issues which
  require a global response.
- Tobacco smoking, the major personal behaviour affecting health, has
  received much epidemiological attention; the tobacco induced epidemics
  continue unabated.
- HIV/AIDS, the most devastating of the new communicable diseases, is
  having a major effect on public health, especially in poor countries of
  Africa, and increasingly in Asia.

References

1. Evans RG, Barer ML, Marmor TR. *Why Are Some People Healthy and Others Not?* New York: de Gruyter, 1994.
2. Rose G. *The Strategy of Preventive Medicine.* Oxford: Oxford University Press, 1992.
3. Axelsson G, Liljeqvist T, Andersson L, Bergman B, Rylander R. Dietary factors and lung cancer among men in West Sweden. *Int J Epidemiol* 1996; **25**:32–9.
4. Pearce N, Matos E, Vainio H, Boffetta P, Kogevinas M. *Occupational Cancer in Developing Countries.* Lyon: IARC Scientific Publications, 1994.
5. Powles J. Changes in disease patterns and related social trends. *Soc Sci Med* 1992; **35**:377–87.
6. World Development Report, 1993. *Investing in Health, World Development Indicators.* New York: Oxford University Press, 1993.
7. United Nations Development Programme. *Human Development Report.* New York: Oxford University Press, 1994.
8. UNICEF. *The State of the World's Children.* New York: Oxford University Press, 1995.
9. United Nations Development Programme. *The Human Development Report.* Oxford: Oxford University Press, 1996.
10. World Development Report. *Development and the Environment.* Oxford: Oxford University Press, 1992.
11. Hahn RA, Eaker E, Barker ND, Teutsch SM, Sosniak W, Krieger N. Poverty and death in the United States – 1973 and 1991. *Epidemiology* 1995; **6**:490–7.
12. Dean M. Absolute effects of relative poverty. *Lancet* 1994; **344**:463.
13. Najman JM. Health and poverty: past, present and prospects for the future. *Soc Sci Med* 1993; **36**:157–66.
14. Quick A, Wilkinson RG. *Income and Health.* London: Socialist Health Association, 1991.
15. United Nations Development Programme. *Human Development Report 1995.* New York: Oxford University Press, 1995.
16. Murray CJL, Chen LC. In search of a contemporary theory for understanding mortality change. *Soc Sci Med* 1993; **36**:143–55.
17. Grosse RN. Interrelation between health and population: observations derived from field experiences. *Soc Sci Med* 1980; **14C**:99–120.
18. Halstead SB, Walsh JA, Warren KS (eds). *Good Health at Low Cost.* New York: Rockefeller Foundation, 1985.
19. Caldwell JC. Routes to low mortality in poor countries. *Pop Dev Review* 1986; **12**:171–220.
20. Wilkinson RG. Income distribution and life expectancy. *Br Med J* 1992; **304**:165–8.
21. Watt GCM. Health implications of putting value added tax on fuel: time to combat fuel poverty. *Br Med J* 1994; **309**:1030–1.
22. Kawachi I, Levine S, Miller SM, Lasch K, Amick B. *Income inequality and life expectancy: theory, research and policies.* (Working paper no. 94–2). The Health Institute, New England Medical Center, 1994.
23. Marmot MG, Davey-Smith G. Why are the Japanese living longer? *Br Med J* 1989; **299**:1547–51.
24. Evans RG, Stoddart GL. Producing health, consuming health care. *Soc Sci Med* 1990; **31**:1347–63.

25. Marmot MG, Davey Smith G, Stansfeld S, Patel C, North F, Head J, White I, Brunner E, Feeney A. Health inequalities among British civil servants: the Whitehall II study. *Lancet* 1991; **337**:1387–93.
26. Wennemo I. Infant mortality, public policy and inequality – a comparison of 18 industrialised countries 1950–85. *Sociol Hlth Illness* 1993; **15**:429–45.
27. Smith R. *Unemployment and Health: a Disaster and a Challenge*. Oxford: Oxford University Press, 1987.
28. World Health Organization. *The World Health Report 1995. Bridging the Gaps.* Geneva: WHO, 1995.
29. Watkins K. *The Oxfam Poverty Report*. Oxford: Oxfam, 1995.
30. Davey Smith G. Income inequality and mortality: why are they related? *Br Med J* 1996; **312**:987–8.
31. Horton R. The infected metropolis. *Lancet* 1996; **347**:134–5.
32. Feachem RGA, Kjellstrom T, Murray CJL, Over M, Phillips MA. *The Health of Adults in the Developing World*. New York: Oxford University Press, 1991.
33. Wang'ombe JK. Public health crisis of cities in developing countries. *Soc Sci Med* 1995; **41**:857–62.
34. Heath I. The poor man at his gate. Homelessness is an avoidable cause of ill health. *Br Med J* 1994; **309**:1675–6.
35. World Health Organization. *Water Supply and Sanitation Sector Monitoring Report 1993. Sector status as of 31 December 1991*. Geneva: WHO/UNICEF, 1993.
36. McMichael AJ. *Planetary Overload. Global Environmental Change and the Health of the Human Species*. Cambridge: Cambridge University Press, 1993.
37. Vidal J. Ready to fight to the last drop. *Guardian Weekly*, August 20th, 1995.
38. World Health Organization. *Diet, Nutrition, and the Prevention of Chronic Disease. Technical Report Series No. 797*. Geneva: WHO, 1990.
39. Barker DJP. *Fetal and Infant Orgins of Adult Disease*. London: British Medical Journal, 1992.
40. Brown L. *Vital Signs*. New York: WW Norton, The World Watch Institute, 1994.
41. Hetzel BS. From Papua New Guinea to the United Nations: the prevention of mental defect due to iodine deficiency. *Aust J Publ Hlth* 1995; **19**:231–4.
42. Adams TAI. International Council for Control of Iodine Deficiency Disorders, and the Hetzel phenomenon. *Aust J Publ Hlth* 1995; **19**:225.
43. Evans I. SAPping maternal health. *Lancet* 1995; **346**:1046.
44. Caldwell C. Health transition: The cultural, social and behavioural determinants of health in the third world. *Soc Sci Med* 1993; **36**:125–35.
45. Green M. Air pollution and health. Not a crisis, but action is needed. *Br Med J* 1995; **1995**:401–2.
46. Hong CJ. Personal communication. Global burden of diseases from air pollution. Geneva: WHO, 1996.
47. Bobak M, Feachem RGA. Air pollution and mortality in Central and Eastern Europe. *Eur J Pub Hlth* 1995; **5**:82–6.
48. Kumar S. Independent assessment at Bhopal. *Lancet* 1994; **343**:283–4.
49. Jasanoff S. *Learning from Disaster: Risk Management after Bhopal*. Philadelphia: University of Pennsylvania Press, 1995.
50. World Health Organization. *Health Consequences of the Chernobyl accident: Results of the IPHECA pilot projects and related national programmes. Summary Report*. Geneva: WHO, 1995.

51. Patz JA, Epstein PR, Burke TA, Balbus, Kornfeld JM. Global climate change and emerging infectious diseases. *JAMA* 1996; **275**:217–23.
52. McMichael AJ, Haines A, Slooff R, Kovat S (eds). *Climate Change and Human Health*. Geneva: WHO, 1996.
53. Myers N, Kent J. *Environmental Exodus: An Emergent Crisis In The Global Arena*. Washington: Project of the Climate Institute, June 1995.
54. Watson RT, Zinyowera MC, Moss RH. *Intergovernmental Panel on Climate Change. Human Population Health. Climate Change 1995: The IPCC Second Assessment Report Vol 2*. Cambridge: Cambridge University Press, 1996.
55. Dyer G. Global warming: it scares the hell out of you. *New Zealand Herald*, December 27th 1995:6.
56. Brack D. Developed world takes the pledge. *Guardian Weekly*, December 31st, 1995:15.
57. McMichael AJ. Contemplating a one child world. *Br Med J* 1995: **311**:1651–2.
58. Anon. Where are the people? *World Health Forum* 1995; **16**:298.
59. Diggory P, Meijer WA, Allbeck R, Black T, Rowley R, Guillehaud J. Legitimate double think. *Lancet* 1993; **341**:1027.
60. Kumar S. India's proposed population policy. *Lancet* 1994; **344**:533.
61. King M. Health is a sustainable state. *Lancet* 1990; **336**:664–7.
62. King M, Elliott C. Double think – a reply. *World Health Forum* 1995; **16**:293–8.
63. Bonneux L. Rwanda: a case of demographic entrapment. *Lancet* 1994; **344**:1689–90.
64. UNICEF. *The State of the World's Children*. Oxford: Oxford University Press, 1992.
65. King M, Elliott C, Hellberg H, Lilford R. Does demographic entrapment challenge the two-child paradigm? *Hlth Pol Planning* 1995; **10**:376–83.
66. Claeson M, Hogan RC, Torres A, Waldman RJ. Double think and double talk. *World Health Forum* 1994; **15**:382–5.
67. McIntosh CA, Finkle JL. The Cairo Conference on population and development: a new paradigm? *Pop Dev Review* 1995; **21**:223–60.
68. Porritt J. Birth of a brave new world order. *Guardian Weekly*, September 11, 1994.
69. Anon. Cairo: a matter of choice. *Lancet* 1994; **344**:557–8.
70. Potts M. USA aborts international family planning. *Lancet* 1996; **347**:556.
71. World Health Organization. *Women, Health and Development. Progress Report by the Director-General*. Geneva: WHO, 1992.
72. Smith R. Overpopulation and overconsumption: combating the two main drivers of global destruction. *Br Med J* 1993; **306**:1285–6.
73. King M, Elliott C. Cairo: damp squib or Roman candle? *Lancet* 1994; **344**:528.
74. World Health Organization. *Tobacco Alert*. Geneva: WHO, July 1995: 2–3.
75. Bartecchi CE, MacKenzie TD, Schrier RW. The human costs of tobacco use. *New Engl J Med* 1994; **330**:907–12.
76. Greaves L. *Smoke Screen. Women's Smoking and Social Control*. London: Scarlet Press, 1996.
77. Graham H. Behaving well: women's health behaviour in context. In: H. Roberts (ed). *Women's Health Counts*. London: Routledge, 1990.
78. Marsh A, McKay S. *Poor Smokers*. Bournemouth: Bourne Press, 1994.
79. Gong YL, Koplan JP, Feng W, Chen CHC, Zheng P, *et al*. Cigarette

smoking in China: prevalence, characteristics, and attitudes in Minhang District. *JAMA* 1995; **274**:1232–4.

80. Yach D. Tobacco in Africa. *World Hlth Forum* 1996; **17**:29–36.
81. Chapman S. All Africa conference on tobacco control. *Br Med J* 1994; **308**:189–91.
82. Chapman S, Richardson J. Tobacco excise and declining tobacco consumption: the case of Papua New Guinea. *Am J Pub Hlth* 1990; **80**:537–40.
83. Townsend J, Roderick P, Cooper J. Cigarette smoking by socioeconomic group, sex, and age: effects of price, income, and health publicity. *Br Med J* 1994; **309**:923–7.
84. Peto R, Lopez AD, Boreham J, Thun M, Heath C. *Mortality from Smoking in Developed Countries 1950–2000: Indirect Estimates from National Vital Statistics*. Oxford: Oxford University Press, 1994.
85. World Health Organization. *Action Plan on Tobacco or Health for 1995–1999*. Manila: WHO Regional Office for the Western Pacific, 1995.
86. World Health Organization. *Tobacco Alert*. Geneva: WHO, January 10, 1995.
87. Rovner J. US tobacco company settles law suit and more. *Lancet* 1996; **347**:823.
88. McCarthy M. US states, tobacco firms, and Medicaid bills. *Lancet* 1994; **344**:253–4.
89. Beaglehole R. Science, advocacy and public health: Lessons from New Zealand's tobacco wars. *J Pub Hlth Pol* 1991; **12**:175–83.
90. Scragg R. A quantification of alcohol-related mortality in New Zealand. *Aust NZ J Med* 1995; **25**:5–12.
91. Rose G, Day S. The population mean predicts the number of deviant individuals. *Br Med J* 1990; **301**:1031–4.
92. Beaglehole R, Jackson R. Alcohol, cardiovascular diseases and all causes of death: a review of the epidemiological evidence. *Drug Alcohol Rev* 1992; **11**:275–90.
93. Lopez A. Personal communication. Geneva: 13 December 1995.
94. McMichael AJ. Vegetarians and longevity: imagining a wider reference population. *Epidemiology* 1992; **3**:389–91.
95. Prentice AM, Jebb SA. Obesity in Britain: gluttony or sloth? *Br Med J* 1995; **311**:437–9.
96. Pate RR, Pratt MP, Blair SN, Haskell WL, Macera CA, Bouchard C, Buchner D *et al*. Physical activity and public health: a recommendation from the Centers for Disease Control and Prevention and the American College of Sports Medicine. *JAMA* 1995; **273**, 402–6.
97. McGinnis JM, Foege WH. Actual causes of death in the United States. *JAMA* 1993; **270**:2207–12.
98. World Health Organization. *Weekly Epidemiological Record (WER) No.27* 5 July 1996, Geneva: WHO.
99. Anon. AIDS spreading like bush fire: education action called for. *New Zealand Herald* December 12, 1995.
100. Montaner JSG, Schechter MT. Time for realism over HIV infection. *Lancet* 1994; **344**:535–6.
101. Anderson JW. India Faces AIDS Explosion. *Guardian Weekly*, 3 September 1995:17.
102. Anon. AIDS: the third wave. *Lancet* 1994; **343**:186–8.
103. Awuonda M. Swedes support UNAIDS. *Lancet* 1995; **345**:1563.

104. Laga M. STD control for HIV prevention – it works! *Lancet* 1995; **346**:518–9
105. Mann J. *Presentation to the Xth International Conference on AIDS*, Yokohama, Japan. August, 1994.
106. Global AIDS Policy Commission. *Towards a New Health Strategy for AIDS*. Cambridge: USA, 1993.
107. World Health Organization. *World Health Organization Report on Road Crashes*. Geneva: WHO, 1989.
108. Mikheev M. New epidemics: the challenge for international health work. In: New Epidemics in Occupational Health. *Finnish Inst Occ Health*, 1994.
109. World Health Organization. *Workers Health Global Medium-term Programme*. Geneva: WHO, 1988.
110. Fontanarosa PB. The unrelenting epidemic of violence in America: truths and consequences. *JAMA* 1995; **273**:1792–3.
111. Anon. Child deaths from gunfire. *New Zealand Herald*, 10 April,1996.
112. Bullock LF, McFarlane J. The birth-weight/battering connection. *Am J Nursing* 1989; **89**:1153–5.
113. Toole MJ, Galson S, Brady W. Are war and public health compatible? *Lancet* 1993; **341**:1193–6.
114. UNICEF. *The State of the World's Children*. New York: Oxford University Press, 1996.
115. Anon. Antipersonnel mines, the all-too-conventional weapon. *Lancet* 1995; **346**:715.
116. Ascherio A, Biellik R, Epstein A, Snetro G, Gloyd S, Ayotte B, Epstein PR. Deaths and injuries caused by land mines in Mozambique. *Lancet* 1995; **346**:721–4.

Part II
Epidemiology

Epidemiology is the study of the distribution and determinants of health related states or events in human populations and the application of this study to the control of health problems. The derivation of the word '*epidemiology*' is Greek: *epi* (upon); *demos* (the people); *logos* (to study). In this part of the book we trace the evolution of epidemiological ideas and methods, assess the achievements and failures of modern epidemiology, and outline the challenges epidemiology will need to confront if it is to assume a more central and constructive position in the health endeavour. An historical focus clarifies the development of epidemiological reasoning and serves to remind us of the early and close connection between epidemiology and the practice of public health.

4

Evolution of epidemiology:
ideas and methods

4.1 Introduction

Epidemiology in its modern form is a relatively new discipline although it has evolved over the last two centuries. The core of epidemiology is the use of quantitative methods to study diseases in human populations so that they might be prevented and controlled. Some of the central ideas of epidemiology extend as far back as the works of the Hippocratic school which emphasised the influence of the physical environment on health over 2000 years ago.

The origins of modern epidemiology can be traced to the work of the English sanitary reformers and French scientists in the first half of the nineteenth century. It emerged as a distinct discipline in the period 1840 70. After a quiescent period at the end of the nineteenth century a revival began in the first half of the twentieth century. The 'modern age' of epidemiology started after the Second World War and since then epidemiology has passed through several phases. It developed in close association with clinical medicine, although because of epidemiology's population-wide focus, this relationship has often been a source of tension. The links between epidemiology and other population sciences, such as demography and the social sciences, have been less well developed.

4.2 The origins of epidemiology

4.2.1 Early origins

Hippocrates, a Greek physician, lived from about 460 to 375 BC. His writings covered a broad range of topics but most of the works attributed to him were, in fact, written by other members of the Hippocratic School; these works are collectively known as the Corpus Hippocraticum. The prime contribution of this school to the evolution of epidemiology was the idea that the environment plays a crucial role in causing disease. Unfortunately the environment was seen in cosmic, astrological or theological terms which were outside the scope of prevention[1]. The Hippocratic school stressed the influence of physical factors on health and disease; for example, variations in weather patterns and the character of the seasons were thought to determine the rise and fall of epidemics[2]. 'Air, Places and Waters' was the first systematic presentation of the relationship between the environment and disease[3]. For more than 2000 years, this was a basic text and provided the theoretical background for understanding disease occurrence (see Box 4.1).

Box 4.1   Hippocrates on 'mode of life'

Hippocrates' comments on the importance of a clean water supply and 'mode of life' are as relevant today as they were 2400 years ago:

Whoever wishes to investigate medicine properly . . . must consider . . . the waters which the inhabitants use, whether they be marshy and soft, or hard, and running from elevated and rocky situations . . . and the mode in which the inhabitants live, and what are their pursuits, whether they are fond of drinking and eating to excess, and given to indolence, or are fond of exercise and labor, and not given to excess in eating and drinking . . .[3].

In his own time, Hippocrates had a strong reputation as a physician and a teacher and the ideas of the Hippocratic School influenced the Greek personal hygiene movement[4]. The Romans also placed great emphasis on public sanitation[5] and many of the conduits built by the Romans remained in use until the early twentieth century. Aqueducts became a symbol of the Roman way of life, as well as a symbol of power. Despite the Greco-Roman emphasis on personal hygiene, life expectancy in this period was only about 25 years and an enormous gap separated the rich and the poor[6]. The ideals promoted by the wealthy citizens had little impact on the general public's health and indeed this was not their purpose.

Following the decline of the Roman Empire in the fifth century, little attention was paid to the science of hygiene, either personal or public. The introduction of Germanic customs in Europe interrupted the Greco-Roman public health tradition until the Christian Mediterranean cities began to expand in the eleventh and twelfth centuries. The physical and economic deterioration and widespread poverty, which followed the decline of the classical civilisations, led to the pandemics of the Middle Ages. This period has been described as a 'universe of hunger' and a 'universe of disease'[7], with a life expectancy of between 30 and 35 years, reducing to about 20 years by the plague pandemic of the year 1348 (Box 4.2).

Box 4.2   Impact of the plague

It was the appearance of the plague in the fourteenth century, and its periodic return throughout the next two centuries, that crystallised the interest in public health that had begun with the isolation of lepers in the thirteenth century[7]. Some cities compiled 'books of the dead' which were comprehensive mortality records used to identify epidemics and follow their course. Mortality rates in the early epidemics were staggering, with up to half of the population dying in cities during the plague pandemic. In response to the first plague pandemic, Northern Italian city-states instituted a series of public health measures designed to protect the health of the elite. For example, the authorities isolated ships suspected of carrying disease; the quarantine lasted for 40 days.

Two main theories of disease – the miasma theory and the contagious theory – competed for centuries. The miasma theory had its origins in the work of the Hippocratic School and was formally developed in the early eighteenth century. A 'miasma', composed of malodorous and poisonous particles generated by the decomposition of organic matter, was thought to be responsible for many diseases. This theory was strongly supported by political and economic groups that sought to avert the imposition of costly quarantine measures justified by the contagious theory of disease. From a practical point of view the miasma theory, although eventually discredited, led to important public health interventions.

The contagious theory was ultimately expressed as the germ theory just over 100 years ago. This theory had its origin in the ancient practice of isolating diseased people and was first stated explicitly by Fracastoro in the sixteenth century. He attributed the spread of epidemics to small 'seeds' which carried the disease. The discovery of micro-organisms with the microscope, invented in 1683, contributed to the development of this theory.

4.2.2 Seventeenth and eighteenth century influences

In the seventeenth century, the foundations of modern clinical medicine were laid by William Harvey and Thomas Sydenham who emphasised the importance of direct observation and experimentation. In parallel, Graunt was laying the basis of health statistics and epidemiology with his analyses of the Weekly Bills of Mortality[8] (Figure 4.1).

The Bills of Mortality were initiated in the late sixteenth century by the parish clerks in London to warn, or reassure, the population about the extent of an epidemic. Using these data, Graunt described patterns of mortality and fertility, for example, the excess of male births, the high infant mortality, and seasonal variations in mortality. Graunt also developed the first life table and proposed that comparisons between countries could be made using this technique. Graunt recognised the limitations of the available data and stressed the need for better data, a continuing concern even today.

Graunt's friend and colleague, William Petty, coined the phrase 'political arithmetic'. This involved the co-ordination of political, economic, social and health surveys to inform public choices and collective action[9,10]. Petty believed that it was in the interests of an economically strong state to have the largest possible number of healthy (and therefore productive) subjects. He wanted to increase the power and prestige of England and, as an essential part of this process, he stressed the need for statistical data on population, trade, manufacture and disease, amongst other topics. Petty's ideas had no immediate effect, in part because of the absence of an effective local civil administration operating under central direction. Modern parallels are not hard to identify.

In 1747 James Lind, a British naval surgeon undertook one of the forerunners of the clinical trial by developing a hypothesis concerning the cause and treatment of scurvy, a debilitating disease now known to be due to vitamin C deficiency[11]. Lind took 12 seamen with scurvy and, in addition to a common diet, gave each of the six pairs a different dietary supplement for 6 days. The two seamen given oranges and lemons made an almost complete recovery. Lind inferred that citric acid fruits cured scurvy and would probably also prevent it. He published his results in 1753, a long delay even by modern publication standards, but it was not until 1795 that the British naval authorities accepted his results and included limes in the diet of sailors. The delay between the original research and its formal application was not due simply to the slowness of the Naval bureaucracy. Of more importance were the difficulties in establishing causality and the general lack of knowledge. Lind's results were not replicated because other theories competed with his. It was not until 1920 that alternative theories were eliminated and agreement reached that scurvy was a dietary deficiency.

In the eighteenth century there was a strong French influence on the

Natural and *Political*

OBSERVATIONS

Mentioned in a following INDEX,

and made upon the

Bills of Mortality.

By *JOHN GRAUNT,*

Citizen of

LONDON.

With reference to the *Government,* *Religion, Trade,*
Growth, Ayre, Diseases, and the several Changes of the
said C I T Y.

——— *Non, me ut miretur Turba, laboro,*
Contentus paucis Lectoribus ———

L O N D O N,
Printed by *Tho: Roycroft,* for *John Martin,* *James Allestry,*
and *Tho: Dicas,* at the Sign of the *Bell* in St. *Paul's*
Church-yard, MDCLXII.

Figure 4.1. Bills of Mortality.

development of epidemiology through the work of mathematicians such as Laplace. The repressive political climate resulted in a reluctance in France to link statistical theory with social and political reality as advocated by Petty[9]. The dominant theory of disease in eighteenth century France stressed the importance of natural phenomena such as climate[12]. The French Revolution stimulated a general interest in public health, initiated the Parisian School of Medicine, and encouraged the epidemiological approach to disease by symbolising a break with past traditions[13]. This approach was also used in China following the 1949 revolution.

4.2.3 The nineteenth century blossoming

The industrial revolution had a profound effect on the health of populations. The squalor and poverty associated with urbanisation provided a direct threat to the health of the labour force and therefore an economic and political threat to industrialists and politicians. The appalling social conditions stimulated the interest of reformers who gradually realised the power of statistical data.

The growth of statistical ideas during the nineteenth century was intimately related to the growth of epidemiology. Major epidemiological developments occurred as a result of the tutelage of Pierre Charles Alexander Louis in Paris in the middle years of the nineteenth century. Louis' ideas were spread to England by Farr, Budd and Guy (the author of the first book on public health[14]), and to the United States of America by many clinicians including Holmes and members of the Shattuck family.

Louis was the first to introduce statistics to medicine and he did more than anyone else in the nineteenth century to develop the central concepts of epidemiological methods and reasoning. He also integrated philosophical and quantitative concepts and applied them to the study of disease, the so called 'methode numérique'. Almost singlehandedly he initiated the period of 'statistical enlightenment', although there was strong opposition from many of his colleagues who feared that statistical methods would obscure the importance of individual variations[15]. A well-known contribution by Louis was the demonstration of the harmful effects of routine bleeding. Ironically Louis' ideas, although enthusiastically taken up by public health practitioners, had little impact on medical practice until the development of clinical epidemiology over a century later[16].

The early years of the nineteenth century in France were also the creative period of the French Hygienist's movement. The climatic theory of the causation of disease yielded to a theory based on the importance of social and economic causes of disease. This approach was epitomised by the work of René Villerme who extensively studied the living conditions and health of Parisiens. As the industrial revolution developed, this led to the investigation of occupational diseases[12]. Occupational studies have continued as a major focus of epidemiology, especially of the occupational risks for cancer[17].

One hundred years after Lind's experiment, an important series of comparative studies were conducted by Semmelweiss on mortality from puerperal fever in two Divisions of the Lying-In hospital in Vienna (see Box 4.3).

Box 4.3 An early clinical trial

Semmelweiss identified the contagious nature of puerperal fever by comparing mortality rates between 1841 and 1846 in the Division staffed by physicians and their assistants, who came to the maternity wards after attending autopsies, and in the Division used for training midwives. Semmelweiss hypothesised that the high maternal mortality in the Division staffed by physicians resulted from the transmission of infectious particles from the autopsy room to the maternity ward. In 1847 he introduced handwashing with a chlorinated solution by the physicians and their assistants before they performed deliveries; the death rate fell immediately to the level of that in the Division staffed by midwives:[11]

| | Physician's division | | | | Midwives's division | | |
| | | Deaths | | | | Deaths | |
Year	Births	No.	%		Births	No.	%
1842	3287	518	15.8		2659	202	7.5
1844	3157	260	8.2		2956	68	2.3
1846	4010	459	11.4		3754	105	2.7
Introduction of intervention (handwashing) in May 1847							
1848	3556	45	1.3		3219	43	1.3

It is ironic that after about 1850 French epidemiology declined, just at the time that epidemiology was growing vigorously in England on the basis of the work of Louis' students. The decline of epidemiology in France has been attributed to the absence or non-utilisation of vital statistics which in England date back to the Bills of Mortality[13]. The development of epidemiology in the United States of America, 40 years later than in England, was due to the time it took Louis' students to develop vital statistical systems in the United States.

The other ingredients necessary for the blossoming of epidemiology were present in all three countries: an identifiable philosophy of epidemiology; a familiarity with statistics; and a well-organised hygienic movement. It is interesting to draw parallels with the continuing poor state of epidemiology in some affluent European countries, such as Germany, which is due, in part, to the lack of access by epidemiologists to vital statistics. A worrying trend in many countries is the conflict between 'individual rights' and the 'common good' which is reflected in the development of privacy laws to further restrict this access.

In both England and France there was a close connection between epidemiology and the public health movement in the nineteenth century. This connection provided a major stimulus to epidemiology[18]. The work of the sanitary physicians (so called because they earned their livelihood by clinical practice) and the organisation they began, the London Epidemiological Society, led to the formal creation of the discipline of epidemiology. In 1863 the term 'scientific epidemiologists' was used, the first known reference to 'epidemiologists'[19].

The credit for institutionalising epidemiology in England is due to William Farr who built on the ideas of Graunt and Petty. Farr acquired an interest in health statistics when studying with Louis in Paris. In 1839 he was appointed to the newly established General Register Office where he initiated an anatomically based system of vital statistics which is the basis of the International Classification of Diseases, now in its tenth revision. Over the next 40 years Farr developed methods for studying the distribution and determinants of human diseases.

Farr's contributions cover the broadest range of epidemiological methods and many are still in use (see Box 4.4). He was not only one of the founders of modern epidemiology, he was also one of the leaders of the public health movement. Farr had a firm commitment to environmental reform using medical and political ideals to reinforce each other[20]. Farr saw statistics as the science of social reform, a science which gave reformists a focus and a platform for a limited range of social reforms, mainly educational and sanitary[21]. In many respects, epidemiologists have lost this commitment to ensuring that epidemiological data is used for reform purposes.

For Farr, human health was a prerequisite to social advancement. He believed that the State had a responsibility to prevent poverty, but he also reflected the ambivalence of many middle class reformers towards poverty. On the one hand was the moralistic view which blamed the poor for their

Box 4.4   Weekly reports in the 'spirit of Farr'

In 1960 the 'spirit of Farr' was revived in the Morbidity and Mortality
Weekly Reports published by the Communicable Disease Center in Atlanta,
Georgia[22]. Many countries are now issuing regular surveillance reports, all
of which bear some resemblance to Farr's reports, and the World Health
Organization publishes the Weekly Epidemiological Record. A recent
example from WHO shows the pattern of deaths due to haemorrhagic fever,
in the Bandunu Region, Zaire, between April and June 1995[23].

Figure 4.2 traces the rise and fall of deaths from Ebola haemorrhagic fever
epidemic in mid-1995 in Zaire. In total, 315 cases occurred with 244 being
fatal.

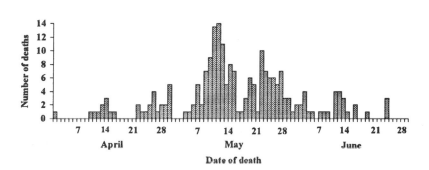

Figure 4.2. Ebola haemorrhagic fever epidemic in mid-1995 in Zaire.
Source: WHO (ref. 23).

own misery and opposed public support for the poor. On the other hand,
Farr had a genuine sympathy for the 'worthy' poor. In this view poor relief
was necessary both to protect the poor and to secure social order. Despite
the complexity and often contradictory nature of Farr's views about the
nature and causes of poverty, he concluded that public intervention was
part of the solution[21]. His vision was broad: 'No variation in the health of
the states of Europe is the result of chance; it is the direct result of the physical and political conditions in which nations live' – a statement which
remains as true today as it was in 1866.

Farr stressed the need for economic, environmental and social reforms to
improve health. Chadwick, one of Farr's contemporaries, reached different
conclusions. He believed that disease aggravated poverty and increased the
costs of supporting the poor. Chadwick brought together a mass of

information in 1842 in the 'Report on an Inquiry into the Sanitary Conditions of the Labouring Population of Great Britain'. As a result, the General Board of Health was created in 1848 with responsibility for public health, but it lasted only seven years.

The broad approach of the sanitary movement was gradually replaced by more specific ideas concerning, for example, the importance of clean water. Notable studies were carried out by John Snow, one of the founders of modern epidemiology and a contemporary of Farr. He investigated, in an integrated series of studies, the causes of the cholera epidemics of 1848–49 and 1853–54. Snow is most remembered for his identification of the Broad Street pump as the vehicle for an explosive epidemic in Soho in August–September 1854[24]. Snow's investigations were brilliant, systematic, thorough, and wide ranging and his later studies were based on a prior hypothesis concerning the contagious nature of cholera[25]. He described the epidemiology of the cholera epidemic in a social and economic context and was much more than a narrowly focused quantitative epidemiologist, as he is usually portrayed in epidemiological texts[26]. In the first decade after Snow's initial publication, little credence was given to the drinking water theory of the origin of cholera. His work did not achieve the status of a 'classic' until after the reprint of his original work in 1936[27].

Guy and Farr became closely associated with the Statistical Society of London which had been founded in 1834. By the mid-nineteenth century, this Society was the centre of biostatistics and epidemiology and was involved with five major statistical areas, including medical statistics. During the 1840s, epidemiology began to emerge as a separate discipline but the application of epidemiological approaches to disease control remained unco-ordinated until 1850[19]. In this year, the London Epidemiological Society was founded to inform the medical profession, the public and politicians about the raging epidemic of cholera. The meetings of the London Epidemiological Society marked the foundation of modern epidemiology and the society flourished during the next 20 years (Box 4.5).

The Society withered with the death of its founding members. Its demise marked the end of the first epidemiological era and was replaced by the bacteriological era from about 1870. For the next half century, epidemiology was overshadowed by the bacteriological paradigm in which laboratory based criteria for judging causal relationships, the Henle-Koch postulates, replaced the population based inferences of the mid-nineteenth century epidemiologists[20]. It was only in the early decades of the twentieth century, when it became apparent that bacteria were not responsible for all diseases, that epidemiology gradually reappeared. In comparison with other health

Box 4.5 The London Epidemiological Society[19]

The purposes of the London Epidemiological Society were:

to institute rigid examination into the causes and conditions which influence the origin, propagation, mitigation, and prevention of epidemic disease . . . to institute . . . original and comprehensive researches into the nature and laws of disease . . . to communicate with government and legislature on matters connected with the prevention of epidemic diseases . . . to publish original papers; to issue queries; to publish reports; to form statistical tables; to prepare illustrative maps; and to collect works relative to epidemic disease.

Comparative mortality studies, evaluations of smallpox inoculation and vaccination, and morbidity surveys were frequently carried out. Most of the work was performed by clinicians acting as epidemiologists in a part-time and unpaid capacity. *The Journal of Public Health* was founded in 1855 and published the transactions of the London Epidemiological Society until 1859 when it was discontinued for financial reasons.

sciences, the consolidation of epidemiology as a flourishing discipline was delayed by almost a century. Epidemiology was initially intimately concerned with promoting and protecting the public's health. Unfortunately modern epidemiologists have neglected this tradition, to the detriment of the public's health. This tradition needs to be reclaimed.

4.3 The twentieth century resurgence

4.3.1 Non-communicable disease epidemiology

During the period dominated by bacteriology, biostatistics continued to develop under the leadership of Galton and Pearson and departments of statistics nourished the next generation of epidemiologists. Foremost among them were Major Greenwood and Percy Stocks in England, and Wade Hampton Frost in the United States of America, all of whom combined the disciplines of biostatistics and epidemiology and were concerned with both infectious and non-infectious diseases. In 1935 Greenwood published 'Epidemics and Crowd Disease', with chapters on tuberculosis and other infectious diseases, but also on cancer and psychological causes of illness[28]. The appointment of Ryle as the first Professor of Social Medicine at Oxford University in 1943, symbolised the emerging importance of non-infectious disease epidemiology. Bradford Hill, initially a colleague of Greenwood, introduced the numerically naive medical profession to the facts of statistical life in a series of articles which were subsequently reprinted in book form[29].

Research in non-communicable disease epidemiology in Great Britain developed primarily as an academic discipline whereas in the United States of America it was based, at least initially, in Departments of Health: federal, state and local. In both countries, occupational studies remained an important focus of epidemiology. The Hygienic Laboratory, established by the United States Public Health Service in 1887, was involved in both infectious and non-communicable disease epidemiology. Goldberger, working for the Hygienic Laboratory, identified the cause of pellagra through an elegant series of studies conducted between 1914 and 1930. He demonstrated that pellagra was not an infectious disease, as was generally believed, but the result of a dietary deficiency later found to be nicotinic acid, part of the vitamin B complex. In the 1930s, important epidemiological studies of fluoride and dental disease were conducted, culminating in a community-based experiment in Grand Rapids, Michigan. In 1946 the Communicable Disease Center was founded by conversion of the agency for Malaria Control in War Areas and provided federal support and leadership for epidemiology; later it became the Centers for Disease Control[30]. The Epidemiologic Intelligence Service of the Centers for Disease Control trained many physicians in the methods of infectious disease epidemiology.

The influence of the health transition in refocusing the task of epidemiology towards non-communicable disease cannot be overemphasised. The increase in death rates from age related diseases, such as heart disease and cancer, caught the attention of epidemiologists. Initially, these diseases were thought to be degenerative in origin, that is, an inevitable consequence of the ageing process. A major outcome of the early studies of lung cancer and heart disease was to shift attention to the role of potentially preventable environmental causes. This marked a dramatic shift from the dominance of the early infectious disease paradigm. Infectious disease epidemiology remains important in wealthy countries because of the emergence of new infectious diseases, such as AIDS, and the re-emergence of 'old' diseases such as tuberculosis, and in poor countries because of the continuing epidemics of infectious diseases.

Evidence for the emergence of a new epidemiological paradigm is to be found in the systematisation of the epidemiological literature, the concentration in wealthy countries on non-communicable diseases, the development of graduate training programmes, and the availability of research funds[31]. The shift in focus from a search for specific infectious agents to the search for multiple causes led, in the space of a few decades after the Second World War, to the development of a wide range of methods and to the maturation of epidemiology[31]. The practice of epidemiology encouraged the development of epidemiological theory and methods, mostly by statisticians.

The transition from infectious to non-communicable disease epidemiology occurred smoothly, at least in part because the technical differences between the divisions are minor and arbitrary[32]. Although the natural histories of the two broad groups of disease are often different, both infectious and non-infectious diseases can be acute or chronic. Tuberculosis was the bridging condition for many epidemiologists making the transition from the study of infectious to non-communicable diseases.

There are several reasons for the early emergence of non-communicable disease epidemiology in Great Britain and the United States of America, but not in Germany, Scandinavia, France or Eastern Europe. The central role of a system of vital statistics was critical, although such systems were well developed in Scandinavia. The strong tradition of an independent epidemiological discipline in Great Britain was also important. The establishment of public health institutions, such as the London School of Hygiene and Tropical Medicine and the schools of public health and research institutes in the United States, fostered interdisciplinary groups of epidemiologists and biostatisticians and, in the United States, provided a major new source of research funding. Many of these new institutions were established with the support of the Rockefeller Foundation and played a role in supporting the process of colonisation in Africa and Asia.

The success of the new paradigm was ensured by the outcome of two research endeavours begun in the late 1940s. Firstly were the results of case control studies in the United States of America and Britain linking cigarette smoking with lung cancer[33,34], even if not all scientists, let alone politicians, accepted the findings[35]. Secondly was the Framingham study, a cohort study initially of heart disease, which was soon expanded to study a wide range of non-communicable diseases and now includes the children and grandchildren of the original cohort[36].

4.3.2 *Phases of modern epidemiology*

Since 1946 there have been several phases in the development of epidemiology. The whole period has been called the 'second epidemiologic revolution' or the conquest of non-communicable diseases, in contrast to the 'first

epidemiologic revolution', which focused on the conquest of infectious diseases[37]. It is now apparent that the conquest of infectious diseases is far
from complete and is unlikely ever to finish[38–40]. What is now required is a
third 'epidemiological revolution' which integrates methods for the study
and control of infectious and non-communicable diseases and examines
their common causes and solutions from a global perspective.

The first phase of modern epidemiology, from 1946 to the mid-1960s, saw
the creation of epidemiological methods necessary for the study of non-
communicable diseases, including methods for estimating various measures
of risk. The publication in 1960 of the first text on modern epidemiology
was a critical point in the evolution of epidemiology[41]. This text contained
the first systematic discussion of epidemiological study designs and the first
explicit mention of the multi-causal web of causation which has dominated
epidemiology[42].

Another early textbook listed the 'personal characteristics' with which
the epidemiologist is primarily concerned: demographic, biological, socioeconomic, and personal living habits[43] By focusing on the agent, host and
environment as the principal determinants of disease occurrence, the social
system became sidelined and it has largely remained outside the consideration of epidemiologists.

The second phase from the mid-1960s to the early 1980s covered the development of more sophisticated methods including the clarification of bias
and confounding, interaction, and the practical development of the case
control study design. The development of computers enhanced methods of
analysis, especially of large data sets. The publication in 1983 of the first
edition of Last's Dictionary of Epidemiology[44] represented an important
consensus on epidemiological terminology, including a widely accepted definition of epidemiology itself, something which had eluded previous generations of epidemiologists[45]. The dictionary is now in its third edition[46]
indicating the continuing evolution of epidemiological terminology.

The third phase, over the last decade, has emphasised the coherence of
epidemiological study designs and the unitary nature of epidemiological
methods, irrespective of the subject matter[47]. Greater attention has been
given to the measurement of exposure which had previously taken second
place to the measurement of outcomes. A large range of exposures is now
studied in the epidemiology of non-communicable diseases. In the 1980s,
and judging from papers published in the *American Journal of
Epidemiology*, aspects of diet, use of tobacco and alcohol, occupation, past
medical history, and use of medications were the most commonly studied
exposures[48].

'Molecular epidemiology', the use of biological markers as more precise indicators of exposure effect, susceptibility or outcome, has generated considerable interest, especially in cancer epidemiology[49]. Molecular techniques may overcome the limited ability of epidemiology to elucidate mechanisms; molecular epidemiology holds the promise of opening the 'black box' of epidemiology and exploring intervening pathways and causal processes[16,50]. The demonstration of the person to person tracking of HIV and tuberculosis are good examples of the potential contribution of molecular epidemiologists[51]. This approach, however, has so far yielded few new hypotheses and has contributed little of substance to benefit the public's health[52]. There is a real danger that the molecular paradigm will come to dominate epidemiology in the same way as the germ theory achieved dominance at the end of the nineteenth century.

Experimental epidemiology has, over the last decade, gained greater status and methods of aggregating and summarising data from numerous small studies are now common. The most recent topic to engage epidemiologists has been the impact of global environmental changes on health. This area will make fundamentally new demands on the practice of epidemiology, as we shall see in Chapter 6.

A feature of epidemiological practice has been the subdivision of the discipline into various branches which describe the type of exposure (e.g. nutritional, environmental or occupational epidemiology), or disease (e.g. cancer, cardiovascular disease or injury epidemiology), or group of participants under study (e.g. paediatric or clinical epidemiology), and even more inappropriately, the technique used (e.g. molecular epidemiology). It would be more appropriate for the subspecialities to become united under the label of 'public health epidemiology', as distinct from 'clinical epidemiology'[53]. There has also been a division among epidemiologists in their sphere of interest, between those interested in the health problems of wealthy countries and those more interested in poor countries[54].

4.4 Ideas and methods

Epidemiology is unique because of its way of looking at problems, its theories and methods, and the problems it studies – states of health and disease in human populations. The central ideas of epidemiology are relatively simple, and many have been known since the time of William Farr in England and Louis in France 150 years ago[19].

There are two fundamental types of epidemiological ideas:

- causal inference, that is, the identification of causal pathways; and
- theoretical and methodological issues related to study design and analysis.

The major recent improvements in epidemiology have been in the areas of study design and analysis.

4.4.1 Causal inference

The early literature on causal inference was systematised by Hill in 1965[55]. The origin of Hill's criteria can be traced back to the eighteenth century Scottish philosopher David Hume[56]. The United States Surgeon General, in assessing the association of smoking with lung cancer in 1964, described five criteria for judging the causality of a given association. This early literature emphasised that causal inference required qualitative judgements based on the available quantitative evidence. This necessity for exercising judgement is often held against epidemiologists by other biomedical scientists and politicians with both groups, when it suits them, requiring 'certainty'.

The criteria proposed by Hill (see Box 4.6) were neither all necessary, apart from temporality, nor sufficient, and have continued to generate much criticism, especially from scientists more familiar with laboratory techniques. Hill cautioned against the unthinking use of hard rules, and while appreciating that all scientific work is incomplete, recognised the need

---

Box 4.6   Criteria for causation as proposed by Hill[55]

Strength	What is the strength (relative risk) of this association?
Consistency	Has the association been 'repeatedly observed by different persons, in different places, circumstances, and times'?
Specificity	Is this association limited to 'specific workers and to particular sites and types of disease'?
Temporality	'Which is the cart and which the horse'?
Biological gradient	Is there a dose-response curve?
Plausibility	Is the association biologically plausible?
Coherence	'The cause-and-effect interpretation should not seriously conflict with the generally known facts of the natural history and biology of the disease'.
Experiment	Is there experimental, or semi-experimental, evidence?
Analogy	Is it 'fair to judge by analogy'?

to act on existing knowledge. The criteria, which have since been revised, are mutually supportive and complementary[57].

Over the last two decades a more formal approach to causality has been encouraged by Popper's view of the central role of falsifiability in science[58]. In this view, causal inference results in a much more tentative conclusion because it is based on the exclusion of other causes for the observed association. This view, however, can lead to a retreat into purity and away from reality. Discussions over the value and meaning of Popper's ideas continued for over a decade and contributed to a broader philosophical inquiry on the nature of the discipline. One important outcome of the Popperian debate is the recognition that epidemiology is concerned with much more than data gathering and is not simply a set of methods.

In part, the usefulness of Popper's ideas depends on the purpose of epidemiology. As pure scientists, epidemiologists can remain tentative about the nature of associations. As public health specialists, however, judgements must be made in the absence of final proof in order to reduce the health risks to the public. Unfortunately, this distinction sets up a dichotomy and can lead to the divorce of epidemiology from its purpose – the prevention and control of disease. The Popperian debate has now faded without having left much impact on the practice of epidemiologists; epidemiologists are now free to again rediscover the social context of their work.

4.4.2 Study design

The development of epidemiological study designs and methods went hand in hand. The unified nature of epidemiological study designs is now increasingly recognised with the randomised controlled trial promoted as the 'gold standard'[47]. When modern epidemiology began to mature at the end of the 1940s, the cross-sectional survey, adapted from the social sciences, was the major study design. As the weaknesses of the survey become apparent, particularly as a tool in the search for causation, more complex and robust designs become popular. Surveys continue to have an important role in assessing the health status of populations and have become institutionalised in many countries. In general, surveys remain more popular with other social scientists than with epidemiologists.

4.4.2.1 Cohort studies

The Framingham Study was the prototype of the longitudinal or cohort study. It was established to measure incidence rates of heart disease in the general population but soon expanded to examine factors influencing the development of heart disease. The Framingham Study has been very influential, yet as originally conceived, the study would not have received funding support through the current peer review system. The aims were poorly addressed, the required sample size was not specified, data collection methods were not described, and the reliability of the data not assessed. Despite these weaknesses, now so apparent in retrospect, the study was a powerful force in shaping the development of epidemiology.

The Framingham Study led to other cohort studies, both of cardiovascular and other non-communicable diseases, and to long-term community studies. The classic cohort study is both more expensive and more time consuming than other study designs. The historical cohort study and the nested case control study have been developed to make economical use of the advantages of the cohort designs.

The modern form of the cohort study combines two features: simplicity of design and large size, often in specific and convenient occupational groups. The Nurses' Health Study, for example, collected baseline information by mailed self-administered questionnaires from approximately 120 000 married nurses in the north eastern states of the United States of America[59]. Mortality is assessed from the national vital registration system and self-reported morbidity is validated on a subsample. The generalisability of results from this type of 'convenience' cohort is dependent on confirmation by other studies. New cohort studies have recently been promoted in several poor countries mainly to document the size of tobacco attributable mortality[60], although this is a questionable use of limited research resources.

4.4.2.2 Case control studies

Case control studies now dominate epidemiology, especially in North America. This design was for many years treated with scorn by epidemiologists raised on the cohort design. Case control studies are relatively cheap to perform in comparison with cohort studies and large randomised controlled trials, and have advantages for the study of diseases with a long interval between exposure to the possible cause and the onset of disease, as the starting point for this study design is cases with established disease. This design avoids the need for the long periods of follow-up required in all but the largest cohort studies.

The antecedents of the case control study lie in the clinical case series and several of these early studies included information on non-cases to provide a reference for comparison of various exposures[61]. Gregg, for example, compared the frequency of a history of rubella in cases of congenital cataract and 100 other patients attending his clinic in the early 1940s[62].

The modern use of the case control design began with the studies on smoking and lung cancer in the United States of America and Britain[33,34], the latter, in particular, laying out the essential features and potential problems of the design. Remarkable developments and extensions of the case control design have occurred and texts are now devoted solely to this design[63]. There is now a sound appreciation of the potential sources of bias to which this method is prone, especially in the selection of controls, and of methods for its avoidance. This study design has been used to assess the efficacy of health service interventions, for example screening. In the so called 'case crossover study', the case acts as it own control where short-term exposures are under investigation.

4.4.2.3 Experimental studies

The best study design for hypothesis testing is the experimental design. Because of the time and effort involved, however, as well as ethical issues, the use of this design is limited. It is particularly suited for the assessment of the value of medical treatment where clear hypotheses can be tested. The antecedents of experimental studies in epidemiology can be traced back to Lind's study of treatment for scurvy in 1753[11]. The importance of comparative studies of medical therapies has long been recognised. Although Fisher introduced randomisation into agricultural research in the 1920s, random allocation of participants was introduced into medical research by Bradford Hill only in 1946. Prior to the initial Medical Research Council trials, various other forms of allocation had been used including alternation, whereby alternative participants were allocated to different arms of the trial[64]. Hill was also responsible for stressing the importance of the analysis of randomised controlled trials on the basis of 'intention to treat'.

The modern era of clinical trials began with the multi-centre trial of streptomycin in the treatment of tuberculosis conducted for the Medical Research Council in Britain in the late 1940s[65]. Streptomycin, a new drug for the treatment of tuberculosis, was available in sufficient quantities for only about 50 patients. The trial gave impressive results; after six months treatment with streptomycin and bed rest, seven of 55 patients were dead, compared with 27 of 52 patients who received only bed rest. On the basis of this trial, streptomycin was accepted as standard treatment for tuberculosis, although the problem of drug resistance was soon recognised. The experimental design has also been used to great effect in the study of preventive interventions. An early randomised controlled trial tested the value of a pertussis vaccine[66]. Other examples include the assessment of the BCG vaccine for tuberculosis and the poliomyelitis vaccine.

Since 1985 about 40 000 randomised controlled trials have been published[67]. Increasingly, randomised controlled trials are undertaken in poor countries or in poor populations with high mortality and morbidity. Unfortunately the results are not always applicable to the populations from which the study participants are drawn. Health services in poor countries may not be suitable for the delivery of the intervention if, in fact, it is shown to be useful. In most of the world, health budgets are woefully inadequate and may not be sufficient or flexible enough to include new interventions or treatments. These considerations should be explored well before studies are conducted in all settings, but they are especially important in poor countries.

Major experimental studies have not always produced clear answers and the results have often generated controversy, particularly when behaviour modification has been the focus. For example, the Multiple Risk Factor Intervention Trial failed to demonstrate an effect on total mortality of several interventions against coronary heart disease in high risk middle aged men in the United States of America[68]. The outcome of this trial is open to several interpretations and its policy implications are not clear. A particular difficulty faced by this trial, and the more recent large scale cardiovascular disease community intervention projects, is the striking decline in cardiovascular disease mortality in the United States of America. This decline has reduced the chance of detecting a reduction in mortality in the treatment group (or community) because of the general reduction in risk factor levels reflecting the success of population wide prevention efforts.

In contrast, large scale, simple and collaborative randomised controlled trials of the treatment of common conditions have on occasions influenced physician behaviour in a relatively short time. For example, the ISIS-2 study of the separate effects of streptokinase and aspirin on survival after acute myocardial infarction involved over 17 000 patients in Western Europe, North America and Australasia[69]. Each drug was found to reduce the case fatality by about 20% and the two combined reduced it by about 40%. Prior to this massive study, many small trials had been completed with mixed results and only about 5% of cardiologists in the United Kingdom were routinely using streptokinase. After the results of the ISIS-2 trial and another similar trial in Italy[70] were published, it was shown that 95% of cardiologists were routinely using both streptokinase and aspirin in appropriate patients[71].

The mega-trials of necessity do not always adhere to all the principles of good study design; for example, they are not always double blind and informed consent from participants is not always possible. Furthermore, huge trials on poorly defined groups of patients may not provide the detailed information required in clinical practice to ensure the best therapy for specific groups of patients[72]. The results of trials on highly selected patients may also be of little use to practising physicians dealing with a wide range of patients under routine conditions. At the other end of the spectrum, randomised controlled trials in single patients, so called 'n of 1 trials', have been used when there is doubt about the best treatment for a stable condition in individual patients[73].

4.4.2.4 Ecological studies

The emphasis on within population study designs has led to the neglect of studies focusing on the major, and largely unexplained, differences between populations in disease rates. Ecological studies address these population differences by examining the relationship between average disease rates and average exposure levels among populations that are often defined geographically. This design is simple and easy to apply and has been used to good effect in exploring interpopulation differences in health status. Because of the population wide focus, this design offers much potential for public health and the results of many ecological studies have endured[74]. Unfortunately this design has until recently been a relatively unsophisticated tool, prone to bias. The ecologic study design does not link outcome events to individual exposure at the level of the individual, and this is the source of their special biases; the 'ecologic fallacy' results from the fact that the average exposure of a group of people does not necessarily reflect their individual risk[75]. The evaluation of bias in ecologic studies is especially difficult because of the many potentially interacting variables that may differ across geographical regions. This study design has been very useful for identifying hypotheses which can be tested with more robust designs and recent methodological work has increased the value of this type of study[74,76].

4.4.3 Epidemiological analyses

A critical development, which began with a paper published in 1946[77], has been the attention given to systematic sources of error (bias) in epidemiology. In 1979, Sackett identified over 35 potential sources of bias[78]. For practical purposes they can be grouped into three major categories: selection, misclassification, and confounding, although confounding is not now generally regarded as a bias, but as a particular feature of the data under investigation.

Estimation of risk, both relative and absolute, is central to epidemiology and was first discussed formally in 1951[79]. Methods of adjusting estimates of risk for possible confounding were developed[80] and have become increasingly sophisticated. Furthermore, the crude risk rate has been broken down into two components, one reflecting confounding and the other reflecting the effect of the exposure[81]. The central importance of obtaining valid results for all studies, irrespective of their design, is now appreciated, as is the fact that even randomised controlled trials are subject to bias.

An unfortunate legacy of the input of statisticians into the development of epidemiological methods has been the dominance of statistical hypothesis testing in data analysis, at the cost of meaningful interpretation. Fortunately, this approach is increasingly being replaced by alternative methods that emphasise estimation of the strength of associations. Statisticians also developed multivariate models in epidemiology to overcome the problems generated by limited data in the ordinary stratified analysis. The first multivariate model was used by Cornfield in his analysis of data from the Framingham study[82]. The multiple logistic model method has now become a primary tool of epidemiology. The rapid advance in computers has encouraged the practical and, often unthinking, application of a range of multiple logistic methods; there is still much to be gained from simpler methods of cross-classification, a point often lost on those who are seduced by powerful computer programmes.

The important effect of sample size on statistical power is now recognised and, in retrospect many early studies, especially clinical trials, produced false negative results as a consequence of insufficient sample size. This recognition has led to large and rather simple randomised controlled trials (the 'mega-trials') and to the overviews or meta-analyses (statistical pooling) of data from numerous small trials investigating the same issue; guidelines for improving meta-analysis have been developed[83]. The hallmark of the modern overview, which is gradually replacing reviews based on the opinions of experts, is that it is undertaken according to strict statistical criteria. The procedure requires that all properly conducted trials are included, irrespective of whether they have been published. A major impediment to systematic overviews is that about half of the 40,000 trials published since 1985 are not retrievable by expert Medline searches[67,84]. The quantitative results of the overview provides a good indication of the effect that could be expected in a similar group of patients; many useful overviews are now influencing clinical practice. The Cochrane Collaboration has been initiated to further the practice of meta-analysis and the dissemination of its results[67].

4.5 Conclusion

The basic notions of epidemiology have their origin in the works of the Hippocratic School which, over 2000 years ago, stressed the importance of the environment for health. The origins of modern epidemiology go back only to the early decades of the nineteenth century. Two historical themes are of continuing importance: the strong statistical contribution to the development of epidemiology and the original and close connection between epidemiology and public health practice.

Non-communicable disease epidemiology had its origins in the years following the Second World War when studies were initiated into the causes of two modern epidemics: heart disease and lung cancer. Over the last four decades, epidemiology has made important contributions to our understanding of the causes of both communicable and non-communicable diseases. Few of these advances rival the contribution of the early, and in retrospect, rather simple studies of the adverse health effects of tobacco. Technical aspects of epidemiology have developed remarkably over the last two decades and the discipline has more and more concentrated on methods, rather than ends.

Epidemiology has contributed greatly to improving the health of populations worldwide. If epidemiology is to fulfil its potential, however, it will need to address several challenges which are described in the next two chapters.

Chapter 4   Key Points

- Epidemiology in its modern form developed over the last half century in response to the emergence of non-communicable disease epidemics.
- Recent developments include mega-trials and meta-analyses.
- Epidemiology has concentrated on studies of individuals and neglected the largely unexplained differences in disease rates between populations.
- Epidemiology has increasingly concentrated on technique and is losing its connection with public health practice.

References

1. Stallones RA. To advance epidemiology. *Ann Rev Public Health* 1980; **1**:69–82.
2. Rosen G. *A History of Public Health*. Baltimore and London: Johns Hopkins University Press, 1958.
3. Hippocrates. *The Genuine Works of Hippocrates*. Translated from Greek by Francis Adams. Baltimore: Williams and Wilkins, 1939.
4. Nutton V. Healers in the medical market place: towards a social history of Graeco-Roman medicine. In: Wear A (ed.). *Medicine in Society*. Cambridge: Cambridge University Press, 1992.
5. Winslow CEA. *Man and Epidemics*. Princeton: Princeton University Press, 1952.
6. Carmichael AG. History of public health and sanitation in the West before 1700. In: Kiple KF (ed.). *The Cambridge World History of Human Disease*. Cambridge: Cambridge University Press, 1993.
7. Park K. Medicine and society in Medieval Europe, 500–1500. In: Wear A (ed.). *Medicine in Society*. Cambridge: Cambridge University Press, 1992.
8. Rothman KJ. Lessons from John Graunt. *Lancet* 1996; **347**:37–9.
9. White KL. *Healing the Schism. Epidemiology, Medicine, and the Public's Health*. New York: Springer, 1991.
10. Banta JE. Sir William Petty: modern epidemiologist (1623–1687). *J Comm Hlth* 1987; **12**:185–98.
11. Lilienfeld AM. Ceteris paribus: the evolution of the clinical trial. *Bull Hist Med* 1982; **56**:1–18.
12. Hannaway C. Discussion (The French influence on the development of epidemiology – Lilienfeld DE and AM). In: Lilienfeld AM (ed.). *Times, Places, and Persons: Aspects of the History of Epidemiology*. Baltimore: Johns Hopkins University Press, 1980.
13. Lilienfeld AM, Lilienfeld DE. *Foundations of Epidemiology*. New York: Oxford University Press, 1980.
14. Guy WA. *Public Health: A Popular Introduction*. London: Renshaw, 1874.
15. Lilienfeld DE, Lilienfeld AM. The French influence on the development of epidemiology. In: Lilienfeld AM (ed.). *Times, Places, and Persons: Aspects of the History of Epidemiology*. Baltimore: Johns Hopkins University Press, 1980.
16. Vandenbroucke JP. Epidemiology in transition: a historial hypothesis. *Epidemiology* 1990; **1**:164–7.
17. Pearce N, Matos E, Vainio H, Boffetta P, Kogevinas M. *Occupational Cancer in Developing Countries*. Lyon, International Agency for Research on Cancer, 1994.
18. Lilienfeld AM, Lilienfeld DE. Epidemiology and the public health movement: a historical perspective. *J Pub Hlth Pol* 1982; **3**:140–9.
19. Lilienfeld DE. The greening of epidemiology: sanitary physicians and the London Epidemiological Society (1830–1870). *Bull Hist Med* 1979; **52**:503–28.
20. Susser M, Adelstein A. The work of William Farr. In: M Susser. *Epidemiology, Health & Society*. New York: Oxford University Press, 1987.
21. Eyler JM. The conceptual origins of William Farr's epidemiology: numerical methods and social thought in the 1830s. In: Lilienfeld AM (ed.). *Times, Places, and Persons. Aspects of the History of Epidemiology*. Baltimore: Johns Hopkins University Press, 1980.

22. Langmuir AD. William Farr: founder of modern concepts of surveillance. *Int J Epidemiol* 1976; **15**:13–18.
23. World Health Organization. *Weekly Epidemiological Record*. Geneva: WHO, August 25, 1995.
24. Winkelstein W. A new perspective on John Snow's communicable disease theory. *Am J Epidemiol* 1995; **142**:S3–S9.
25. Vandenbroucke JP. Which John Snow should set the example for clinical epidemiology? *J Clin Epidemiol* 1988; **41**:1215–16.
26. Cameron D, Jones IG. John Snow, the Broad Street pump and modern epidemiology. *Int J Epidemiol* 1983; **12**:393–6.
27. Vandenbroucke JP, Eelkman Rooda HM, Beukers H. What made John Snow a hero? *Am J Epidemiol* 1991; **133**:967–73.
28. Greenwood M. *Epidemics and Crowd Diseases: An Introduction to the Study of Epidemiology*. London: Williams and Northgate, 1935.
29. Hill AB. *Principles of Medical Statistics*. London: Lancet, 1937.
30. Terris M. Healthy lifestyles: the perspective of epidemiology. *J Pub Hlth Pol* 1992; **13**:186–94.
31. Susser M. Epidemiology in the United States after World War II: the evolution of technique. *Epidemiol Rev* 1985; **7**:147–77.
32. Barrett-Connor E. Infectious and chronic disease epidemiology: separate and unequal? *Am J Epidemiol* 1979; **109**:245–9.
33. Wynder EL, Graham EA. Tobacco smoke as a possible etiologic factor in bronchiogenic carcinoma: a study of 654 proved cases. *JAMA* 1950; **143**:329–36.
34. Doll R, Hill AB. Smoking and carcinoma of the lung: preliminary report. *Br Med J* 1950; **ii**:739–48.
35. Vandenbroucke JP. Those who were wrong. *Am J Epidemiol* 1989; **130**:3–5.
36. Dawber T. *The Framingham Study*. Cambridge: Harvard University Press, 1980.
37. Terris M. The complex tasks of the second epidemiologic revolution: the Joseph W. Mountin Lecture. *J Pub Hlth Pol* 1983; **4**:8–24.
38. Berkelman RL, Hughes JM. The conquest of infectious diseases: who are we kidding? *Ann Intern Med* 1993; **119**:426–7.
39. Hughes JM, La Montagne JR. Emerging infectious diseases. *J Infect Dis* 1994; **170**:263–4.
40. Epstein PR. Emerging diseases and ecosystem instability: new threats to public health. *Am J Pub Hlth* 1995; **85**:168–72.
41. MacMahon B, Pugh TF, Ipsen J. *Epidemiologic Methods*. Boston: Little Brown and Co, 1960.
42. Krieger N. Epidemiology and the web of causation: has anyone seen the spider? *Soc Sci Med* 1994; **39**:887–902.
43. Lilienfeld AM. *Foundations of Epidemiology*. New York: Oxford University Press, 1976.
44. Last JM. *A Dictionary of Epidemiology*. New York: Oxford University Press, 1983.
45. Lilienfeld DE. Definitions of epidemiology. *Am J Epidemiol* 1978; **107**:87–90.
46. Last JM. *A Dictionary of Epidemiology*, 3rd edn. New York: Oxford University Press, 1995.
47. Rothman K. *Modern Epidemiology*. Boston: Little Brown & Co, 1986.
48. Armstrong BK, White E, Saracci R. *Principles of Exposure Measurement in Epidemiology*. Oxford: Oxford University Press, 1992.

49. McMichael AJ. 'Molecular epidemiology': new pathway or new travelling companion?'. *Am J Epidemiol* 1994; **140**:1–11.
50. Susser M, Susser E. Choosing a future for epidemiology: 1. Eras and paradigms. *Am J Pub Hlth* 1996; **86**:668–73.
51. Wilcox AJ. Molecular epidemiology: collision of two cultures. *Epidemiology* 1995; **6**:561–2.
52. Pearce N, de Sanjose S, Boffetta P, Kogevinas M, Saracci R, Savitz D. Limitations of biomarkers of exposure in cancer epidemiology. *Epidemiology* 1995; **6**:190–4.
53. Mackenbach JP. Public health epidemiology. *J Epidemiol Comm Hlth* 1995; **49**:333–4.
54. Wall SGI. Epidemiology in developing countries. *Scand J Soc Med* 1990; **Suppl. 46**: 25–32.
55. Hill AB. The environment and disease: association or causation? *Proc R Soc Med* 1965; **58**:295–9.
56. Morabia A. On the origin of Hill's causal criteria. *Epidemiology* 1991; **2**:367–9.
57. Susser M. What is a cause and how do we know one? A grammar for pragmatic epidemiology. *Am J Epidemiol* 1991; **133**:635–48.
58. Susser M. The logic of Sir Karl Popper and the practice of epidemiology. *Am J Epidemiol* 1986; **124**:711–18.
59. Colditz GA, Bonita R, Stampfer MJ, Willett WC, Rosner B, Speizer FE, Hennekens CH. Cigarette smoking and risk of stroke in middle-aged women. *New Engl J Med* 1988; **318**:937–41.
60. World Health Organization. *Tobacco Alert*. Geneva: WHO, January 10, 1995.
61. Armenian HK, Lilienfeld DE. Overview and historical perspective. *Epidemiol Rev* 1994; **16**:1–5.
62. Gregg NM. Congenital cataract following German measles in the mother. *Trans Ophthalmol Soc Aust* 1941; **3**:35–46.
63. Schlesselman JJ. *Case-Control Studies: Design, Conduct, Analysis*. New York: Oxford University Press, 1982.
64. Doll R. Sir Austin Bradford Hill and the progress of medical science. *Br Med J* 1992; **305**:1521–6.
65. Medical Research Council Streptomycin in Tuberculosis Trials Committee. Streptomycin treatment for pulmonary tuberculosis. *Br Med J* 1948; **ii**:769–82.
66. Medical Research Council Whooping-cough Immunisation Committee. The prevention of whooping-cough by vaccination. *Br Med J* 1950; **i**:1463–71.
67. Godlee F. The Cochrane Collaboration. *Br Med J* 1994; **309**:969–70.
68. MRFIT (Multiple Risk Factor Intervention Trial Research Group). Mortality rates after 10½ years for participants in the Multiple Risk Factor Intervention Trial. Findings related to a prior hypothesis of the Trial. *Circulation* 1990; **82**:1616–28.
69. ISIS-2 Collaborative Group. Randomised trial of intravenous streptokinase, oral aspirin, both, or neither among 17 187 cases of suspected acute myocardial infarction. *Lancet* 1988; **ii**:349–60.
70. GISSI. Effectiveness of intravenous thrombolytic therapy in acute myocardial infarction. *Lancet* 1986; **i**:397–401.
71. Doll R. Development of controlled trials in preventive and therapeutic medicine. *J Biosoc Sci* 1991; **23**:365–78.
72. Ertl G, Jugdutt B. ACE inhibition after myocardial infarction: can megatrials provide answers? *Lancet* 1994; **344**:1068–9.

73. Guyatt G, Sackett D, Adachi J, Roberts R, Chong J, Rosenbloom D, Keller J. A clinican's guide for conducting randomised trials in individual patients. *Can Med Assoc J* 1988; **139**:497–503.
74. Susser M. The logic in ecological: II. The logic of design. *Am J Pub Hlth* 1994; **84**:830–5.
75. Greenland S, Robins J. Ecologic studies: biases, misconceptions, and counterexamples. *Am J Epidemiol* 1993; **139**:747–60.
76. Susser M. The logic in ecological: I. The logic of analysis. *Am J Pub Hlth* 1994; **84**:825–9.
77. Berkson J. Limitations of the application of fourfold table analysis to hospital data. *Biometrics* 1946; **2**:47–53.
78. Sackett DL. Bias in analytic research. *J Chron Dis* 1979; **32**:51–63.
79. Cornfield J. A method of estimating comparative rates from clinical data. Applications to cancer of the lung, breast, and cervix. *J Natl Cancer Inst* 1951; **11**:1269–75.
80. Mantel N, Haenszel W. Statistical aspects of the analysis of data from retrospective studies of disease. *J Natl Cancer Inst* 1959; **22**:719–48.
81. Miettinen OS. Components of the crude risk ratio. *Am J Epidemiol* 1972; **96**:168–72.
82. Cornfield J. Joint dependence of risk of coronary heart disease on serum cholesterol and systolic blood pressure: a discriminant function analysis. *Fed Proc* 1962; **2**:58–61.
83. Sackett DL, Spitzer WO. Guidelines for improving meta-analysis. *Lancet* 1994; **343**:910.
84. Dickersin K, Scherer R, Lefebvre R. Identifying relevant studies for systematic reviews. *Br Med J* 1994; **309**:1286–91.

5

The current state of epidemiology: achievements and limitations

5.1 Introduction

Many of the historical epidemiological achievements have already been referred to in earlier chapters. In this chapter we review the current state of epidemiology, summarising some of the recent achievements and concentrating on the limitations of the epidemiological methods and outlook. The chapter also reviews some of the main criticisms of epidemiology. The next chapter continues this theme and identifies the main challenges facing epidemiology. Some epidemiological achievements can also be viewed as failures, and many achievements are not the sole responsibility of the epidemiologists involved. Nevertheless, it is useful to attempt to summarise the state of epidemiology, fully recognising that other reviewers might come up with different conclusions – a timely warning on the perils of reviews!

5.2 Achievements

5.2.1 The growth of epidemiology

Epidemiology is flourishing in many countries. The 'fall' of epidemiology by the year 2000, predicted by Rothman in 1981[1], now seems most unlikely, judging by the proliferation of peer reviewed journals, the lively discussion of epidemiological methods and results in medical journals, and its popularity with the media. There is a worrying trend, however, at least in the United States of America, for young epidemiologists to withdraw from the field[2].

Despite the overall growth of epidemiology, there is both a global shortage and a maldistribution of epidemiologists, reflecting poor workforce planning[3]. It is difficult to estimate the required number of epidemiologists. Should they rank on a per capita basis with general practitioners, brain surgeons or sociologists? A feature of the discipline, especially in North America, has been the increase in non-physician epidemiologists. In 1975 there was no more than 500 fully trained epidemiologists in the United States of America, 300 of whom were physicians[4]; by 1985 there were an estimated 4600 epidemiologists, 54% of whom were physicians[5]. By the year 2000 it is suggested that the United States of America will require about five times the 1990 number of medically trained epidemiologists[4].

There is little information on the gender and ethnic composition of the epidemiological workforce. A 1992 study by the American College of Epidemiology found a severe under-representation of minority groups in epidemiology, especially in relation to the severity of the ethnic morbidity and mortality gap. For example, in 1992 African-Americans, who made up 12% of the population, constituted only 2% of epidemiology faculty members in epidemiology degree programmes. There was also a marked deficit of students from minority population groups[6].

When compared with other public health disciplines within the United States of America (biostatistics, health services administration, health education and environmental sciences), epidemiology had the second lowest level of minority representation amongst faculty and the lowest among students[7]. Faculty representation of minority groups in public health in the United States of America was virtually unchanged between 1985 and 1992, although the percentages of students from minority groups increased by more than one-third during this period, largely because of increases in Hispanic and Asian students[7].

It is a sad irony that epidemiology which has exposed the health impact of social disadvantage, now find its own ranks less socially representative than other public health disciplines. Recommendations have been made to improve the participation of under-represented minority group in epidemiology[6]. It is to be hoped that epidemiology can rapidly improve its own 'health'; to this end, the American College of Epidemiology has produced a statement of principles which recognises the importance of achieving racial and ethnic diversity in the profession[8].

The situation of epidemiology in poor countries is even more difficult to assess. In 1994 the International Epidemiological Association had a total of 2237 members, including 156 in Africa, 127 in South East Asia, 83 in the Eastern Mediterranean region and 132 in South American countries[9]. It is not known how well these numbers reflect the active epidemiological workforce and many epidemiological studies in poor countries are conducted, at least in part, by epidemiologists based in wealthy countries; this type of epidemiology produces its own challenges, both practical[10,11] and ethical[12], and its own rewards[13].

In summary, epidemiology has flourished in some countries; however, there is a global shortage of epidemiologists, an under-representation of minority groups, and a maldistribution of the available workforce.

5.2.2 *Epidemiology and health status: essential but not sufficient*

Epidemiology has undoubtedly contributed directly to global improvements in health. For example, without the contribution of epidemiologists small pox would not have been eradicated or the health hazards of tobacco identified in such (excruciating) detail. Epidemiology has identified the causes of many non-communicable diseases and contributed to their prevention, including heart disease and stroke, and dietary deficiency diseases such as iodine deficiency. Two recent contributions are the identification of the probable causes of an iatrogenic epidemic of death from asthma[14] and of sudden infant deaths[15]. Infectious disease epidemiologists have made many contributions and take credit, most recently, for our understanding of the AIDS epidemic, despite our inability to act on this knowledge to prevent the global spread of AIDS.

With regard to cancer there has been debate as to whether the so called 'war against cancer' is being won or lost. A decline in mortality has been noted for most, but not all, cancers. Lung cancer has already outstripped breast cancer mortality in women in the United States of America. For most cancers in children and young adults, mortality rates are declining[16]. Of those cancers in which incidence rates have increased substantially since the early 1970s, one is associated with the spread of AIDS (Kaposi's sarcoma) and two may be due to more frequent screening (breast and prostate). Only for lung cancer, testicular cancer and melanoma are the increases in incidence rates independent and genuine. These favourable trends in cancer incidence and mortality indicate the importance of epidemiology and prevention, because only a small amount of the improvement is due to specific treatments, for example, leukemia, especially in young people.

Unfortunately, the relationship between epidemiological endeavour and health improvements is not always clear. Although it is relatively easy to identify the contribution of epidemiology to the control of specific diseases over the last few decades, it is much more difficult to assess the contribution of epidemiology to the dramatic overall improvement in health status over the last century. As epidemiology is only one part of public health, and public health is only one of the factors contributing to health improvement, this is not surprising.

In assessing the value of epidemiology to health improvements, the case of tobacco is instructive. The case control studies published in 1950, now viewed as epidemiological classics, were the first of literally thousands of studies of this association. In the absence of epidemiological data, the cause of the epidemics of lung cancer and other tobacco induced diseases could not have been identified. This knowledge has been an essential stimulus for public health action. By itself, however, knowledge is not sufficient to promote adequate control measures. Where progress has occurred, a constellation of forces has acted together[17]. Despite over four decades of research and public health intervention, more people are now exposed to, and die from, tobacco than ever before. Research interventions in wealthy countries which have focused on consumption and not production, have only added to the inequalities in health between the poor and rich within wealthy countries, and between poor and wealthy countries.

A similar focus on the adverse effect of consumption of a high fat diet on cardiovascular disease and educational efforts directed towards encouraging knowledge of personal cholesterol levels, has also contributed to widening social class differentials in coronary heart disease occurrence in wealthy countries. Health education strategies have too often focused on modification of individual risk factors to the neglect of the commercial forces which encourage consumption of fat. As a consequence, while educated and relatively wealthy people have been able to reduce their cardiovascular disease risk status, poor people have been less successful. Furthermore, the consequences of the animal-oriented agriculture business which supports the mass consumption of saturated fat has been almost entirely neglected[18].

5.2.3 *Contributions to medical care*

Epidemiology has also made important contributions to the medical care of individuals through the application of the randomised controlled trial to medical care issues[19], studies of the effectiveness and efficiency of health services, and the development of 'clinical epidemiology' and its new incarnation, 'evidence-based medicine'[20].

The Cochrane Centre was established in Oxford in 1993 to facilitate systematic and up-to-date reviews of randomised controlled trials of health care. Information from the Centre, which maintains a register of systematic reviews and randomised controlled trials (both published and unpublished), is disseminated through seminars, workshops and electronic media including the 'Online Journal of Current Clinical Trials'. The Centre encourages the formation of collaborative review groups which may be problem-based (e.g., coronary heart disease, stroke, breast cancer, pregnancy and childbirth), intervention based (e.g., nutrition, neonatal care), or speciality based (e.g., public health, primary care). The collaboration is limited to randomised studies and thus will not be useful for the many areas which are not appropriate for randomised trials, for example, some preventive interventions such as suicide prevention[20].

The importance of systematic overviews and dissemination of results is readily illustrated. The first trial of the use of corticosteroids by women for the prevention of respiratory disease in potentially premature babies was published in 1972[21]. It was not until 1989, however, that a systematic review of the many, usually small, randomised controlled trials in this area demonstrated that corticosteroids reduced by 30 to 50% the risk of babies dying from the complications of immaturity[22]. Many obstetricians would not have been aware until the 1989 review was published of the benefits of this form of care. In retrospect, enough information was available ten years earlier for the evidence to change practice.

Clinical epidemiology has generated controversy. Some see it as a contradiction in terms[23]; others view it as outdated, a threat to health, or as a part of a movement serving the interests of pharmaceutical companies[24,25]. There is no doubt that the application of epidemiological methods and principles to medical practice has been of benefit, despite this being remarkably slow. Advice contained in medical textbooks and review articles often fails to reflect the strong evidence available from randomised controlled trials thus delaying implementation of some life-saving therapies[26]; other treatments continue to be recommended long after controlled trials have shown them to be either ineffective or even harmful.

Regrettably, epidemiology, and public health more generally, have had little impact on debates on the reorganisation of health services which are occurring in most countries. Powerful vested interests and ideological considerations are much more influential in directing or resisting changes to the organisation and delivery of health services. For example, the recent debate about the reform of health care in the United States of America has not been led by public health practitioners[27]. It is thus not surprising that when health services are re-organised (or 'redisorganised'), the focus is not on public health.

5.3 Limitations

Epidemiology has been criticised from two different perspectives representing different philosophies and different conceptions of health and disease: the individualistic and the collectivist[28]. The individualistic view emphasises the primacy of the individual; society, in this view, is the outcome of the actions and motives of distinct individuals. In the collectivist view, the emphasis is on society as a whole. The individualistic philosophy has its counterpart in the natural science or mechanistic view of health which underpins modern medicine and considers health as the absence of disease. The contrasting broad view of health is enshrined in the original WHO definition of health.

Most of the criticism of epidemiology is based on the mechanistic view of health and concentrates on the supposed failure of epidemiology to reach the standards of other natural sciences. Concern has been expressed at the epidemiological emphasis on risk factors for multi-factorial diseases, on the poor quality of epidemiological data, and on a general failure to adhere to 'scientific standards'. More challenging criticisms of epidemiology have been expressed from the broad population perspective[18,29,30]. The most immediate threat to epidemiology is that posed by the mechanistic critics as they challenge the ability of epidemiology to meet 'scientific' criteria.

5.3.1 'Risk factor' epidemiology

Critics are justified when they point to the loose use of the term 'risk factor', and the equation of risk factors with causes[31,32]. Many critics are unable to separate important risk factors from the trivial associations that so much delight the mass media, and do not use the techniques and criteria available for exactly this purpose. While it is counterproductive to dismiss all risk factors, it is equally inappropriate to condemn all epidemiological studies of risk factors as unscientific because of a few poor studies. Too often the contributions of this type of epidemiology to our understanding of the causes of the cardiovascular disease and cancer epidemics are ignored; furthermore, epidemiological studies of high quality often lead to appropriate biological research[33].

The multi-factorial concept of disease is a useful reflection of the real world. Some critics are convinced that non-communicable disease epidemiology is stagnating and believe that further understanding of coronary heart disease, for example, will come from laboratory studies and not from epidemiology, despite the impressive gains from prevention over the last two decades[34]. The causes of the major differences in disease experience within and between countries, however, will not be discovered in a laboratory.

One persistent critic of 'risk factor' epidemiology (also referred to as 'black box' epidemiology) went further and questioned the raison d'être of epidemiology[31,35,36,37]. Skrabanek asserted that epidemiologists turned their attention away from infectious diseases (because these diseases were becoming less prevalent) leaving an epidemic of epidemiologists who are short of diseases suitable for study[31]. In part this is true; of much more importance, however, was the rise in death rates from non-communicable diseases. Skrabanek believed that the preoccupation with causes and prevention of disease encouraged epidemiologists to become moralists, preaching the 'good life'[31].

Two examples used to illustrate the 'poverty of epidemiology' are amylnitrate as a cause of AIDS and the association of oestrogen replacement therapy with heart disease in women[35]. To the credit of epidemiology, the amylnitrate and AIDS relationship was soon discarded as a hypothesis when HIV was discovered[38]. The conflicting results of two studies published in the same issue of the *New England Journal of Medicine* on the associations of oestrogen replacement therapy with heart disease in women generated controversy and, more importantly, further study[39]. The association of oestrogen replacement therapy with a reduced risk of heart disease is now firmly established. In the absence of randomised controlled trial evidence, however, it is still not clear whether this is a causal association. So, far from indicating epidemiological ineptitude, these studies illustrate the progressive nature of epidemiological research.

5.3.2 Data quality and scientific standards

Epidemiologists have been repeatedly accused of ignoring the common criticisms of epidemiology. These include the use of poor quality data, a lack of precision in measurement, invalid extrapolation, inappropriate use of terminology, bias in the interpretation of data, and an undue emphasis on statistical inference at the expense of causal inference[40-42]. Feinstein is correct in calling for further improvement in the quality of epidemiological data, but there is nothing in this challenge that would not be accepted by most epidemiologists. Indeed, it has been repeatedly identified as a major challenge[43]. There is also support for his call for less dependence on mathematical modelling and the need for epidemiology to become more integrated with other scientific disciplines.

The limitations of their data are all well recognised by most epidemiologists and are addressed through a variety of approaches including the preparation of detailed protocols and manuals of operation. The difficulties in studying human populations explain some of the problems in the science of epidemiology. There is, of course, a need for continuing attention to the scientific quality of the evidence as well as to the appropriate statistical methods of analysis and adjustment[38].

5.3.3 Asocial epidemiology

The most challenging criticisms of epidemiology stem from its individualistic philosophical underpinning and its reluctance to place individuals in their social context[44,45]. In particular, the risk factor approach to epidemiology and prevention does not give adequate weight to the role of social factors in explaining population differences in the distribution of health problems. This individualistic approach also runs the risk of blaming the victim and encouraging health education strategies at the expense of social, economic and environmental changes. The result is the medicalisation of prevention rather than its socialisation. This criticism of epidemiology recognises that the ethics and purpose of epidemiology must be broadened to include the health impact of social, economic and environmental conditions on a range of outcomes, not just death and disease.

It has also been suggested that epidemiology, as it cannot easily tap into the experiences and perceptions of people, is unlikely to be effective when it comes to prevention and control[46]. Epidemiology should combine qualitative studies of the concerns and views expressed by people about the disease or injury under investigation with quantitative information, data gathering and interpretation. Interpretation of both qualitative and quantitative data is critical in understanding what is happening and what can be done.

The aim of epidemiology is to understand the causes of disease so that health status is improved. From this perspective, epidemiology cannot be practised in isolation from the people who make up the study population. Epidemiological studies of the future need to fully integrate qualitative and quantitative research methods in the context of people's lives. The application of this fully rounded approach is most easily envisaged in occupational health epidemiology. It is more difficult to apply in the context of large scale studies of randomly chosen population samples.

Much of the controversy involving and generated by epidemiology is due to the intrinsic imprecision of epidemiology; of more importance is the recent epidemiological emphasis on methods, to the neglect of purpose[18,29]. Ironically, although the distinguishing feature of epidemiology as a science is its population focus, much of modern epidemiology ignores the unique features of populations and instead isolates individual characteristics and risk factors from their social context. The impact of modern epidemiology on public health has been severely limited by this focus on specific individual exposures. The recommended public health interventions have focused on these exposures (risk factors) to the neglect of their social and economic determinants.

The current lack of interest in social factors and the population perspective has been attributed to the personal and professional isolation of epidemiologists who are usually dependent on funding by government or voluntary agencies[47]. The prevailing ideology in most countries now favours individual responsibility over collective responsibility. Unfortunately, for many epidemiologists the study of social factors is considered too political, despite the fact that it is also an implicit 'political' decision not to address the broader issues.

5.4 Conclusion

To its credit, epidemiology survived long neglect at the expense of the bacteriological paradigm. Over the last half century, epidemiology has grown and flourished in many wealthy countries, although there remains an overall shortage of epidemiologists and the workforce is both maldistributed and unrepresentative in ethnic composition. Epidemiology has made many important contributions to the prevention and control of disease, although epidemiology alone cannot claim responsibility for either specific or general health improvements. Epidemiology has contributed to establishing the scientific basis of clinical medicine and has much to offer the health services in the identification of effective and efficient services.

Epidemiology has been criticised from two opposing perspectives. Biomedical scientists are concerned by the inability of epidemiologists to replicate the strict methods of laboratory based science. Social scientists are concerned by exactly this reductionist basis to modern epidemiology; in this view, epidemiology neglects the social context in which people live and work and concentrates on individual attributes at the expense of the characteristics of populations. The 'scientific' criticisms are the most threatening, at least from a funding viewpoint, because the agencies responsible for allocating research funds generally reflect this view. From a public health perspective, the most serious challenge for epidemiology is to re-establish its social responsibility. This is one of several challenges addressed in the next chapter.

Chapter 5   Key Points

* Epidemiology is flourishing, although there is a global shortage of epidemiologists and a maldistribution of the workforce.
* Epidemiology has contributed to the improvements in health status of populations worldwide and to the increased efficiency and effectiveness of medical care.
* Epidemiology has been criticised as being too closely allied with both medicine and the natural sciences and, from another perspective, of ignoring the social and economic determinants of health and disease.

References

1. Rothman KJ. The rise and fall of epidemiology, AD 1950–2000. *New Engl J Med* 1981; **304**:600–2.
2. Harlow BL. Coping with the personal and professional frustrations of epidemiologic research. *Am J Epidemiol* 1995; **142**:785–7.
3. Greenberg RS. The future of epidemiology. *Ann Epidemiol* 1990; **1**:213–4.
4. White KL. Healing the Schism. *Epidemiology, Medicine, and the Public's Health*. New York: Springer, 1991.
5. Williams SJ, Tyler CW, Clark L, Coleman L, Curran P. Epidemiologists in the United States: an assessment of the current supply and the anticipated need. *Prev Med* 1988; **4**:231–8.
6. Schoenbach VJ, Reynolds GH, Kumanyika SK, for the committee on minority affairs of the American College of Epidemiology. Racial and ethnic distribution of faculty, students and fellows in US epidemiology degree programs, 1992. *Ann Epidemiol* 1994; **4**:259–65.
7. Greenberg RS. Is epidemiology broken down by race and ethnicity? *Ann Epidemiol* 1994; **4**:337.
8. American College of Epidemiology. Statement of Principles. *Ann Epidemiol* 1995; **5**:505–8.
9. Noah N. *IEA Database*, Personal communication, October 1994.
10. Fortney JA. Reproductive epidemiologic research in developing countries. *Ann Epidemiol* 1990; **1**:187–94.
11. Taylor PR, Dawsey S, Albanes D. Cancer prevention trials in China and Finland. *Ann Epidemiol* 1990; **1**:195–203.
12. Bonita R, Beaglehole R. Cardiovascular disease epidemiology in developing countries: ethics and etiquette. *Lancet* 1994; **344**:1586–7.
13. Wall SG. Epidemiology in developing countries – some experiences from collaboration across disciplines and cultures. *Scand J Soc Med* 1990; Suppl. **46**:25–32.

14. Pearce N, Beasley R, Crane J, Burgess C, Jackson R. End of the New Zealand asthma mortality epidemic. *Lancet* 1995; **345**:41–4.
15. Mitchell EA, Brunt JM, Everard C. Reduction in mortality from SIDS in New Zealand, 1986–92. *Arch Dis Child* 1994; **70**:291–4.
16. Doll R. Progress against cancer: an epidemiologic assessment. *Am J Epidemiol* 1991; **134**:675–88.
17. Beaglehole R. Science, advocacy and public health: lessons from New Zealand's tobacco wars. *J Pub Hlth Policy* 1991; **12**:175–83.
18. Wing S. Limits of epidemiology. *Med Global Survival* 1994; **1**:74–86.
19. Cochrane A. *Effectiveness and Efficiency*. London: Nuffield Provincial Hospitals Trust, 1972.
20. Godlee F. The Cochrane Collaboration. *Br Med J* 1994; **309**:969–70.
21. Liggins GC, Howie, RN. A controlled trial of antepartum glucocorticoid treatment for prevention of the respiratory distress syndrome in premature infants. *Pediatrics* 1972; **50**:515–25.
22. The Cochrane Collaboration. *Introductory Brochure*. Oxford, 1993.
23. Last JM. What is clinical epidemiology? *J Pub Hlth Pol* 1988; **9**:159–63.
24. Holland W. Inappropriate terminology. *Int J Epidemiol* 1983; **12**:5–7.
25. Terris M. In: Buck C, Llopis A, Napra E, Terris M (eds). *The Challenge of Epidemiology: Issues and Selected Readings*. Washington DC: Pan American Health Organization, 1988.
26. Chalmers I, Haynes B. Reporting, updating, and correcting systematic reviews of the effects of health care. *Br Med J* 1994; **309**:862–5.
27. Navarro V. The future of public health in health care reform. *Am J Pub Hlth* 1994; **84**:729–30.
28. Nijhuis HGJ, Van Der Maesen LJG. The philosophical foundations of public health: an invitation to debate. *J Epidemiol Comm Hlth* 1994; **48**:1–3.
29. Susser M. Epidemiology today: 'a thought-tormented world'. *Int J Epidemiol* 1989; **18**:481–8.
30. McKinlay JB. The promotion of health through planned socio-political change: challenges for research and policy. *Soc Sci Med* 1993; **36**:109–17.
31. Skrabanek P. Risk-factor epidemiology: science or non-science? In: Berger P, Browning R, Anderson D, Skrabanek P, Johnstone JR (eds). *Health, Lifestyle and Environment: Countering the Panic*. London: Social Affairs Unit, Manhattan Institute, 1991.
32. Skrabanek P. Has risk-factor epidemiology outlived its usefulness? *Am J Epidemiol* 1993; **138**:1016.
33. Savitz DA. In defense of black box epidemiology. *Epidemiology* 1994; **5**:550–2.
34. McCormick J, Skrabanek P. Coronary heart disease is not preventable by population interventions. *Lancet* 1988; **ii**:839–41.
35. Skrabanek P. The poverty of epidemiology. *Perspect Biol Med* 1992; **35**:182–5.
36. Skrabanek P. The epidemiology of errors. *Lancet* 1993; **342**:1502.
37. Skrabanek P. The emptiness of the Black Box. *Epidemiology* 1994; **5**:553–5.
38. Vandenbroucke JP, Pardoel VPAM. An autopsy of epidemiologic methods: the case of 'poppers' in the early epidemic of the acquired immunodeficiency syndrome (AIDS). *Am J Epidemiol* 1989; **129**:455–7.
39. Bailar JC. When research results are in conflict. *New Engl J Med* 1985; **313**:1080–1.
40. Stehbens WE. The quality of epidemiological data in coronary heart disease and atherosclerosis. *J Clin Epidemiol* 1993; **46**:1337–46.

41. Feinstein AR. Scientific standards in epidemiologic studies of the menace of daily life. *Science* 1988; **242**:1257–63.
42. Stebhens WE. An appraisal of the epidemic rise of coronary heart disease and its decline. *Lancet* 1987; **i**:606–11.
43. Gordis L. Challenges to epidemiology in the next decade. *Am J Epidemiol* 1988; **128**:1–9.
44. Krieger N. Epidemiology and the web of causation: has anyone seen the spider? *Soc Sci Med* 1994; **39**:887–902.
45. Tesh SN. Miasma and 'social factors' in disease causality: lessons from the Nineteenth Century. *J Hlth Pol, Policy Law* 1995; **20**:1001–24.
46. Arnoux L, Grace V. Method and practice of critical epidemiology. In: Spicer J, Trlin A, Walton JA (eds). *Social Dimensions of Health and Disease: New Zealand Perspectives*. Palmerston North: Dunmore Press, 1994.
47. Pearce N. Traditional epidemiology, modern epidemiology, and public health. *Am J Pub Hlth* 1996; **86**: 678–83.

6

Challenges for epidemiology

6.1 Introduction

The central purpose of epidemiology is the study of epidemics so that they might be prevented and controlled. The main challenges facing epidemiology stem from its two concerns: the scale and nature of human health problems and the desire to improve health. In this chapter we identify several challenges which, if met, will allow epidemiology to flourish in the next century, and will ensure the public's health will receive the full benefit of what epidemiology can offer. This chapter outlines five challenges facing epidemiologists.

6.2 Improving basic epidemiological information

As discussed in Chapter 3, little is known about the global burden of disease and even less about the global distribution of health. Even the most rudimentary data on the number of deaths are missing for much of the world. Methods which estimate the total number of deaths occurring each year provide an indication of the huge global burden of preventable premature death. The information on cause of death is even more scanty and, where it does exist, its validity is often not known. Collecting even the most basic data leads to the recognition of shortcomings which in turn prompt the need for improved information. At a more general level, methods for measuring health status at a population level are seriously deficient. Recent concern about Creutzfeldt–Jakob disease in Europe has highlighted the failure of epidemiology to monitor the occurrence of bovine spongioform encephalopathy[1]. Addressing these gaps is a central challenge facing epidemiologists.

The only readily available information for monitoring international trends in death and disease is the death data provided to the WHO from national vital registration systems, covering about one-third of the world's population. Data on disease incidence and case fatality, which are necessary to understand the reason for mortality trends, are not routinely available. The exceptions are data from cancer registries which are available from 48 cancer registries for approximately 60 populations in 28 countries[2]. These registries require long-term commitment from official agencies and permissive privacy laws.

Information is lacking for the major cause of death worldwide (cardiovascular disease), although a WHO project which is monitoring the trends and determinants of cardiovascular disease (the MONICA Project) will fill the gap for some, mostly European, countries[3]. This project is a result of WHO leadership and has been facilitated by the relative strength of cardiovascular disease epidemiology. The Global Burden of Disease Project has also highlighted the lack of reliable information on the impact of disease on disability[4]; the basic data necessary for assessing this burden is, for the most part, simply not available. In time, this project may produce reliable trend data in a small number of countries. New international collaborations have recently developed to fill gaps in our understanding of the occurrence of diabetes and asthma.

Measuring the burden of disease has not been a priority for epidemiologists, despite the central importance of this task. It is not a glamorous activity and not likely to result in major peer reviewed publications. It is tedious and time consuming and many agencies decline responsibility for its funding. Health research institutions believe it to be a governmental responsibility, and governments in turn accord it a low priority. Furthermore, epidemiologists have not developed methods suitable for the widespread assessment of morbidity. Reliance has been placed on laborious and expensive methods which are barely suitable for ongoing use even in wealthy countries let alone for countries with limited expertise, fewer resources and almost no appropriately trained workforce.

The challenge is to develop and implement cost-effective methods of monitoring the global burden of disease. Traditional methods, involving disease registers and community surveys, are too expensive and cumbersome to be generally applicable. New methods, such as the capture–recapture method offer more promise[5], but require evaluation and testing, especially in poor countries. Information from sentinel sites could easily be aggregated using modern telecommunication networks. There is scope for low cost, but high powered, computer modelling techniques. This type of epidemiological action is not glamorous but should be more actively supported and encouraged by international health agencies.

6.3 Causal inference

There are two aspects to the challenge of determining whether an observed association is likely to be a causal relationship. The first is the need to increase knowledge of causal mechanisms and pathways, focusing especially on the social origins of disease. Much of contemporary epidemiology is guided by the principle that the origins of disease are due to gene–environmental interactions. This 'black box' approach to epidemiology emphasises exposure–disease associations and the idea that disease can be prevented by altering the environment without detailed knowledge of mechanisms[6]. The contributions of this approach have been enormous; one of the best examples is the way smoking was identified as a cause of cancer in the absence of knowledge of mechanisms. Advocates of this approach suggest that a commitment to the search for mechanisms will divert attention from the search for causes.

Some commentators encourage an exploration of the 'black box' of mechanisms so as to avoid epidemiology being swept away, like the miasmists in the twentieth century[7]. This approach fails to acknowledge the history of epidemiology. Indeed, the miasma and the contagion theories are still with us, although neither are in its nineteenth century form. Although the contagious and the environmental approaches are converging, neither approach adequately describes the origin of disease.

A more comprehensive understanding of causal pathways is necessary. For example, although much is known about the causes of coronary heart disease from the level of individual risk factors to the cellular mechanisms in the arterial wall, the huge population differences in risk factor levels are not well understood. The process of causal inference runs the danger of adopting a narrow individualistic focus, and ignoring the social, economic and political contributions to the cardiovascular disease epidemic.

The challenge for epidemiology is to develop sophisticated theories of disease causation that acknowledge the complex social, environmental and economic systems in which the health-disease process is embedded. Various attempts have been made to outline these relationships[8–10], but they are all largely schematic and, as yet, of unproven utility. These models do emphasise the importance of research, however, which places individuals firmly in the context of their social, economic and physical environment. This broad perspective is essential for a fuller understanding of the pathways to health and disease.

The second aspect of this challenge is to deepen understanding of the health transition and the reasons for changing mortality patterns.

Although this transition has long been known to epidemiologists and demographers, efforts to understand the relative roles of contributory factors are rudimentary. Three components of the health transition are described but their relative importance is only guessed at, and our ability to predict the evolution of the ongoing transition is limited. We cannot, for example, be sure as to what will happen to the major non-communicable diseases in poor countries if the transition progresses. The relative contribution of public health and individual medical care to the health transition requires further research.

6.4 Global problems require global solutions

Observers of epidemiology could be excused for thinking that epidemiologists are increasingly concerned with rediscovering and reinforcing the known. The availability of large public domain data sets, the career importance of publications, and the time pressure for producing dissertations, have all encouraged the repetition of safe (and sometimes boring) epidemiological studies. By contrast, the big public health problems have been neglected; the health effects of war, poverty, and global environmental change, have not received the attention they, and the public, deserve.

The potential problems posed by a changing environment have now reached the epidemiological agenda[11]. The problems of war and poverty, although long on the public health agenda, are not a major concern of epidemiologists, most of whom are based in urban centres in wealthy countries. The impact of urbanisation and development on the health transition in poor countries is of critical importance for determining the future global burden of disease. Yet this topic also remains neglected. It is easier to receive research funds to investigate the role of lipoprotein fractions in heart disease, than to explore the burden of disease in poor countries. Epidemiologists must overcome their parochialism and recognise the importance to global health of the disease problems of the poor world.

In part, progress has been slow because of the difficulties in studying the health effects of widespread changes at a global level. New methods and techniques are required as well as new approaches to causal inference, given the complete lack of experimental data and the long time delay between cause and effect. This is a qualitatively different research challenge from ones faced in the past[12]. The emphasis will need to be on prediction rather than estimation and on model building that incorporates other biological data as well as extrapolation from limited empirical data.

More general factors have operated to discourage epidemiologists from dealing with the new global big health problems, most of which are social and economic in origin. The main sources of funding for epidemiological studies are governmental or voluntary agencies which are most supportive of safe and uncontroversial studies of individual risk factors. In turn, this has led to epidemiologists concentrating on research areas which are likely to be funded and which avoid 'political' issues. Furthermore, the study of the big health problems presents enormous difficulties which are outside the traditional skills and techniques of traditional epidemiology and require close collaboration with a range of other disciplines.

The long-term solution to the neglect of the global public health problems is a re-orientation of epidemiology. The big problems will begin to receive the necessary attention when epidemiology returns to being a problem solving discipline, as it was 150 years ago. Noteworthy attempts have been made to deal with the broad health effects of underdevelopment at a population level, not through public health programmes, but by changing the dominant social, economic and political systems, for example in Nicaragua and Chile[13].

The global problems in turn will require the development of new theories, methods and techniques, and not just data; existing study designs are unhelpful when studying, for example, the effects of global warming. Epidemiologists will need to become familiar with, and skilled in, the creative use of new information technologies in the context of a collaborative and inclusive vision of public health in an electronic world[14]. A global agenda for research in epidemiology and public health might help refocus the attention of epidemiologists[15].

6.5 Linking epidemiology and public policy

There are several aspects to the challenge of forging closer links between epidemiology and policy formation.

6.5.1 Building links with policy makers

A most important challenge facing epidemiologists is to develop and strengthen the tenuous link between epidemiological findings and their application. For the last 150 years the justification for epidemiology has been its close connection with public health policy. Epidemiological findings on the causes and prevention of disease always have implications for health policy and public policy more generally. Unfortunately, these implications are not always acted upon.

There are many fine examples of epidemiological results having policy impact, from fluoridation of water supplies and seat belt legislation, to the withdrawal of potentially dangerous pharmaceuticals. There is a vast amount of sound epidemiological information, however, which has not been translated into appropriate policy, and neglected or misinterpreted data abound. Many of the issues studied by epidemiologists are also of great importance to a range of powerful vested interest groups, for example the tobacco and alcohol industries. Perhaps the most striking indictment of the failure to implement epidemiological data is the continuing inaction to prevent the global spread of the tobacco epidemic; the projections of the burden of disease caused by tobacco have done little to halt the spread of this epidemic[16]. Other examples include encouragement of mammographic screening for women under the age of 50 years, despite the evidence showing that it is ineffective in reducing the death rate from breast cancer in younger women; the failure to prevent the global spread of HIV infection despite a decade's knowledge of the means by which the infection is spread; the almost total reliance on the high risk strategy, for example for cardiovascular disease prevention; and the general failure to capitalise on the power of the population strategy for prevention.

There are many reasons for the lack of influence of epidemiology on policy. Many epidemiologists, especially those based in academic institutions, are remote from policy decisions. Some epidemiologists believe in 'pure science'; others believe that their work is 'value free' and should be kept separate from the explicit values of policy. The epidemiological time frame for action is slow and epidemiologists tend to be cautious and pedantic. Yet policy makers often require information at short notice. Epidemiological results are often couched in careful, but ambiguous, terms and sometimes conflicting results emerge which generate debate and confusion. If epidemiologists cannot agree on the meaning of conflicting results, it is easy to see why policy makers will ignore calls for action.

For some epidemiologists remoteness from policy is not an accident, but a conscious choice. There is a view that the science and its policy application should be kept separate, in the interests of maintaining scientific integrity. The editor of the journal *Epidemiology*, for example, discourages authors from linking policy implications with their research finding on the basis that brief discussions of policy, usually at the end of the discussion section of articles, are likely to be facile[17]. This editorial approach which distances epidemiology from its social and policy context is particularly strong in the United States of America and encourages the separation of science from policy. In this view, the only policy role of epidemiologists is as private citizens[18,19]. If epidemiology serves only to study the occurrence of disease and is not involved in prevention and control, then this position is understandable. In our view epidemiologists have an obligation to discuss policy implications which are, after all, the main justification for epidemiology.

The process of influencing health policy and, more generally, public policy, is extraordinarily complex. Epidemiologists are only one rather small group of actors in the process of policy making which balances competing risks and benefits. By informing policy decisions, epidemiology can contribute directly to provide the necessary information to assist in this process, thereby ensuring an improvement in the public's health. Also involved in the policy making process are other scientists, bureaucrats, various professional groups, politicians, and powerful commercial vested interest groups. For many issues, it is only recently that the process of causal inference has become sufficiently developed by epidemiologists for a hypothesis to be supported with enough strength to justify action. Additional reasons for policy ineffectiveness are closely related to several of the other challenges including the isolation of epidemiology from communities, and our inability to develop a comprehensive understanding of the causes of disease.

As with all the challenges to epidemiology, the solution is neither simple nor straightforward. In the first instance, it is necessary for epidemiology to affirm its connection with policy and to reject scientific isolation. More coherent policy advice will arise if epidemiologists work more closely with other social scientists. The policy making process itself requires greater scientific scrutiny. Secondly, epidemiologists and policy makers, irrespective of their background, institutional location or political affiliation, need to establish close links. These links can be based on formal contractual relations or on informal networks. Thirdly, epidemiologists must be exposed in training and in practice to the complexity of policy making. Fourthly, the editorial and peer review process must focus not only on the scientific merit of a paper, but should also encourage discussion of policy implications as is now undertaken, for example, in the *British Medical Journal*. Epidemiological data inevitably illuminates policy options and these should be discussed. Fifthly, grant funding agencies should consider, as one of their criteria, evidence of prior discussions with potential users of the results of the proposed study.

risk communicated !!!

6.5.2 Communicating risk

The process of communicating quantitative estimates of disease risks to the public and policy makers is a serious challenge facing epidemiologists and closely related to the more general challenge of linking epidemiology to public health.

A central task of epidemiologists is the measurement of the strength of observed associations. Various measures of risk are used: relative risk to assess the strength of a relationship; risk differences to measure the impact of the risk factor; and measures of attributable risk to assess the importance of the risk factor from a population perspective.

Almost daily new risks, or 'menaces to daily life', based on epidemiological studies are presented to the public by the media. The proliferation of so called 'health information' allows fatalists to shrug their shoulders and say 'well, what's the point, everything is dangerous', and epidemiology is mocked. Recent examples of small increased relative risks which received media publicity include: passive smoking and heart disease; margarine (*trans* fatty acids) and heart disease; iron and heart disease; abortion and breast cancer; low dose oral contraceptives and pulmonary embolism; and beef eating and the risk of Creutzfeldt–Jakob disease.

Epidemiological findings can be powerful enough to cause epidemics[20]. For example, in 1986, a cancer agency conducted a study of cancer incidence in two suburbs of Edmonton, Alberta, and publicly reported an increase of about 25% over the expected occurrence for most sites of cancer[21]. Residents in these communities had been concerned for several years about an apparently elevated rate of cancer among adults because of the presence nearby of oil refineries and petrochemical factories. Re-analysis of the data several months later revealed an error and correction brought the rates into line with Alberta as a whole. A survey of residents, after realisation of the mistake and before its public correction, studied the response of the communities. The perception of any elevated cancer risk, in the absence of a true risk, had negative effect on the communities, both psychologically and economically.

Another example demonstates that the way in which data from randomised trials are presented significantly influences health policy decisions[22]. For example, the willingness to fund a mammography screening programme (see Box 6.1) was far greater when results of a trial were presented as a relative risk reduction (A) compared with other methods: absolute risk reduction (B), proportion of event free patients (C), or as the number of patients needed to be treated to prevent an adverse event (D).

Box 6.1 Different, but equal, ways of communicating risk[22]

The following four statements based on the results of a randomised
controlled trial of mammographic screening[23] are equivalent.

Over a seven year follow-up period:

A the rate of deaths from breast cancer was reduced by 34%
B the absolute reduction in deaths from breast cancer was 0.06%
C the rate of patients surviving breast cancer was increased from 99.82 to
   99.88%
D 1592 women needed to be screened over 7 years to prevent one death
   from breast cancer

When relative risk estimates are high, communication is easier, but still
not necessarily effective. For example, the relative risk of lung cancer for
a cigarette smoker after 20 years of heavy smoking compared with a
non-smoker is about 20; that is, the heavy smoker has a 20-fold increased
risk of developing lung cancer. In epidemiological terms, this is a very
strong relative risk and most people are aware of this risk, even smokers.
Of course, not every heavy smoker develops lung cancer and the risk is
not instantaneous. Young people, in particular, are more concerned with
immediate social and peer pressures than with long-term risks; and all
smokers can point to a healthy heavily smoking octogenarian. Other
high relative risks are found with exposure to asbestos in association
with smoking, and with some drugs, for example thalidomide in pregnancy.

Most relative risks are an order of magnitude lower, around two, and
increasingly, epidemiologists struggle with the meaning of relative risks in
the range 1.1 to 1.5. The lower the estimate of risk, the more likely it is due
to bias in the design or conduct of the study, especially if it has been found
in only a single study. Although epidemiologists may order their lives on the
basis of quantitative results (less dietary fat, more or less alcohol, more
exercise), most people are more fatalistic, especially young people with
limited social and economic prospects.

The challenge of communicating notions of risk to policy makers and,
even more importantly, to the public, has yet to be seriously contemplated.
The old messages of gloom and doom, so beloved by health educational-
ists, which might be effective for small segments of the population, do not

impact on the great majority of the population. In fact, this type of message contributes to the growing social inequalities in health status within populations.

All epidemiological studies require independent scientific scrutiny and the journal peer review process is not always adequate for this purpose. It is imperative that epidemiologists, peer reviewers and journal editors appreciate the limitations of the data and ensure that the results are presented in a balanced manner, even at the risk of missing media attention. Doll and Hill, in their pioneering studies of smoking and lung cancer set a fine example. When their first study produced an unexpected result (after all they were also interested in the health effects of pollution), further studies were planned which confirmed their original findings. In general, less rush to publication and more discussion and thought will improve communication with the public.

Much more work is required to ensure that epidemiological risks are translated into terms and images that can be readily understood. This is one prerequisite for influencing behaviour. Simple quantitative and probabilistic statements mean little; for example, 'passive smokers have an increased risk of cancer of 30%', oversimplifies a complex epidemiological issue. Statements such as 'each cigarette smoked reduces life expectancy by five minutes' may carry more weight, but this type of message requires testing with smokers of different ages and sex. From a public health perspective, population attributable risk is more important than relative risk; and from a clinical perspective, absolute risk is more important for treatment guidelines. Once the epidemiological data are firm, creativity is required in communicating the appropriate messages in a meaningful manner so that all segments of society benefit.

6.5.3 Overcoming isolation

The isolation of epidemiology from other sciences, public health practitioners, policy makers and the public, limits the ability of epidemiologists to influence policy. There are several aspects to the isolation of epidemiology. Although epidemiologists have usually worked closely with biostatisticians (often out of necessity) collaboration with other public health disciplines such as social scientists, health economists, laboratory based scientists and clinicians has been less obvious. Collaboration with the public is critical.

Part of the problem arises from the separation (or 'schism') between epidemiology and clinical medicine, as in the United States of America, where separate schools of public health were developed in the first half of this century[24]. This separation is also important in countries which have not developed separate public health institutions. For example, even where epidemiology has been located primarily within schools of medicine, as in the United Kingdom, there has been a separation of epidemiology from clinical and laboratory based disciplines.

There is much to be gained from collaboration between epidemiologists with other biological scientists. Findings which may not make biological sense initially may lead to real advances in knowledge. Biological implausibility, however, should alert us to the possibility that epidemiological results have other, more mundane, explanations related to insufficient adherence to basic scientific principles. The distance from biology may be one explanation why distinguished statisticians such as Fisher took a negative position, from a purely statistical viewpoint, on the relationship of smoking to lung cancer[25]. Equally important is the isolation of epidemiology from the full range of social science methods. As a consequence, much of the policy recommendations coming from epidemiology have been one dimensional.

It will not be easy to overcome the isolation of epidemiology from other scientific disciplines. A reorientation and integration of epidemiology teaching with other public health disciplines has enormous potential. Exposure to a broad range of public health disciplines should be mandatory for epidemiology students.

The remedy for the separation of epidemiology from clinical medicine was the development of clinical epidemiology. Clinical epidemiology has taken off in some institutions in wealthy countries, for example at McMaster University in Canada and the University of Newcastle in New South Wales, Australia. The International Clinical Epidemiology Network has been successful in building and supporting the academic public health workforce in several poor countries. Clinical epidemiology has much to offer, both in terms of its potential impact on delivery of health care and also for health service policy. Clinical epidemiology as its name implies, is more important for clinical medicine than for public health and is unlikely to contribute to the development of public health or health policy.

Another aspect of isolation is the separation of academic epidemiology from public health practitioners, especially members of local and central departments of health. A special manifestation of epidemiological isolation, all too common in the United States of America, is the analysis, often by graduate students, of data gathered by someone else. The epidemiological analysis often proceeds in ignorance of the true nature of the data and with a lack of understanding of its strengths and weaknesses. Making connections with public health practitioners to ensure an involvement with public health policy should be a priority for graduate students.

An important and fundamental aspect of the isolation of epidemiologists is that epidemiology is all to often divorced from the public it serves. Only rarely are epidemiological studies designed in close collaboration with representatives of the public. The word 'epidemiology' gives full weight to 'the people' (*demos*). The involvement of the public in epidemiological studies encourages a greater understanding of disease occurrence and is important for a well rounded approach. This involvement is essential, given the paramount importance of social factors in disease. In addition, this approach will facilitate disease prevention because it is based on the experience of people in their own social and economic environments. For example, participatory epidemiology (or 'popular' epidemiology) has developed around the work of toxic waste activists[26]. These activists have created a social movement and have helped to broaden the overall environmental movement. Most often, however, epidemiologists consider the people they study as their 'subjects' or 'patients', though there is now a move to relabel them as 'participants'. Although the labels may have changed, the nature of the relationship is unchanged.

The participation of lay people in popular epidemiology is difficult because of differing conceptions of risk, lack of resources, poor access to information, and unresponsive public health bureaucrats and scientists. Slowly environmental epidemiologists and other public health professionals are recognising and responding to the special challenges of working closely with lay people and their communities[27]. The great attraction of such participation is that it may expand traditional epidemiological approaches to include social and economic factors as part of the causal pathways.

6.5.4 *Achieving breadth and depth*

Modern epidemiology is becoming increasingly concerned with technique[27]. This trend runs the risk of divorcing epidemiology from biology and society giving rise to criticism that it lacks depth and breadth thereby limiting its relevance to public health[28].

This challenge is related to the need to overcome isolation, and it goes beyond the breaking down of barriers. The value of an epidemiological study depends almost exclusively on the hypothesis under investigation which in turn requires well developed epidemiological theories of the social dynamics of health and disease. Epidemiology, however, is much more than

a set of designs and methods. Unfortunately, undue attention in epidemiological teaching is focused on hypothesis testing to the neglect of explicit
theories.

The implicit theory underlying most epidemiology is 'biomedical individualism'. While in practice this involves the exploration of the biological
determinants of disease amenable to medical care, it too often ignores the
social determinants of disease, and treats populations as the sum of individuals. More attention needs to be directed to the creation of productive
and illuminating hypotheses. Much can be learnt from historical examples,
such as the hypotheses concerning scurvy, pellagra, retrolental fibroplasia,
the nineteenth century debate on the relationship of poverty and disease,
and more recently from HIV/AIDS[29].

A good example of the limitation of a narrowly focused epidemiology is
the continuing neglect of the striking impact of social class on the incidence
of disease. Another example is the ongoing concern for identifying the
causes of disease in individuals to the neglect of the causes of a population's
health status. Stressing public health as a prime value will ensure that
research is placed in its social context[30] Multi-disciplinary collaboration
firmly grounded in biology will help develop a creative epidemiology which
is purposeful and focused on the need to prevent and control epidemics.
This will also involve greater concentration on the multiple health outcomes of environmental determinants, rather than working backwards
from a single disease to its multiple causes. From this perspective, cohort
studies are the preferred study design as each case control study can investigate only one outcome.

Creative approaches are also required to ensure that new diseases are
investigated efficiently, irrespective of their origin, utilising a full range of
techniques. Although not the focus of this book, much more creative epidemiology is also required in measuring the effectiveness and efficiency of
health services. Without this creativity, epidemiology will surely become a
'lost cause'.

6.6 The ethical challenge

The final challenge is to ensure that epidemiology reaches and maintains a
high ethical standard. The Helsinki Declaration requires that biomedical
research with humans must conform to accepted scientific principles; it
must be truthful, honest, impartial and objective[31]. Only in the last few
years have epidemiologists seriously considered the ethical implications of
their work[32]. Epidemiologists, along with all other biomedical scientists,

must strive to up hold the four basic principles of biomedical ethics: autonomy, the respect for human rights, dignity and freedom; non-maleficence, the principle of not harming; beneficence, the principle of doing good; and justice, the principle concerned with equity, fairness and truth telling.

Epidemiologists come into conflict with the principles of autonomy and non-maleficence when dealing with the privacy of personal information stored in health records. The protection of personal privacy is, of course, a laudable aim. There is a conflict between this right and the need for research which is in the interest of the 'public good'. Epidemiologists require access to this type of information because ultimately it is in the public interest to use this information to identify new knowledge about the causes of many diseases; strict confidentiality rules must be observed.

By contrast with the potential restriction on epidemiological data, is the much greater freedom allowed journalists[33]. It is a poor reflection on societal values that we are willing to accept journalists' right to invade privacy, but not prepared to protect epidemiological research which is much more in the public interest and less likely to do harm to individuals[34]. There are, in addition, other national threats to epidemiological research. In Germany for instance, access to death certificates and post-mortem reports for research purposes has long been prohibited and psychiatric registers have been closed in both Norway and Germany[33].

A European Union directive on the confidentiality of data balances the rights to privacy with the needs of epidemiological research[35]. This emerged only after an extensive exchange of view points and facts between epidemiologists and legislators. In its original proposal it would have prohibited record linkage studies using existing data sets on the basis that they were unethical[36]; stipulated how long data may could be kept; required written consent before data could be processed; required that the subject of the data should be told about disclosure of data to a third party; and made provision for the the subject's right of access to the data. These requirements would have prohibited observational studies using historical data, for example the studies of Barker and colleagues on the prenatal origins of non-communicable diseases[37]. The original European proposal was potentially so restrictive because it aimed to ensure high and uniform levels of protection.

So far epidemiology has not had to contend with large scale fraudulent investigations although questions have been raised about some data contributed to multi-centre studies of the management of breast cancer in North America[38]. There is an increasing tendency for epidemiological studies to be sponsored by agencies with a direct interest in the association under study. The tobacco industry is notorious in this regard although it now channels research funds through 'independent' trusts. The pharmaceutical industry is now one of the major funders of drug evaluation trials. This type of funding poses enormous ethical problems for epidemiology.

Epidemiological studies in poor countries present particular ethical problems. Western models of science are not universally accepted and epidemiologists working in poor countries may be alienated from the populations studied[39]. Poverty and helplessness is a striking feature of many communities, and not just in the poor world. If communities do not perceive the benefits of epidemiological studies, participation will be low and the community may feel exploited. Randomised controlled trials in poor communities entail additional ethical problems if local health services are poorly organised and health budgets are inadequate to ensure that the local population receives the benefits of the intervention, assuming that it was shown to be effective. Recently attention has also been given to the particular ethics of epidemiology of women's health[40]. For example, the United States Food and Drug Administration in 1993 lifted its ban on including women of childbearing age in early drug trials because of the scientific benefits of their inclusion[41].

The solution to this challenge will depend on how epidemiologists meet the previous challenges. If epidemiology can establish a sound and socially responsible theoretical base and communicate more easily with the public and policy makers, it will be in a more secure position. If at the same epidemiologists accept and adhere to the guidelines proposed by the Council of International Organisations of Medical Sciences (CIOMS), the discipline will rest on a firmer ethical base[42]. Specific guidelines are also required on funding, especially of consultancies, to avoid conflicts of interest. Epidemiologists must not become beholden to vested interests. Researchers sponsored by industry should insist that they retain the right of publication. It is likely that many such studies have been censored by the sponsoring industry, although the extent of this problem is unknown[43]. There is a pressing need for more formal ethics curricula in epidemiological teaching programmes[44].

The issue of advocacy in epidemiology raises important ethical issues. Various ethical guidelines endorse the role of advocate, although the recommendations differ[45]. The guidelines of the International Epidemiological Association recommend separating the roles of scientists and advocates. The CIOMS guidelines recommend advocacy dependent on the quality of epidemiological research and on causal interpretations of the data. The ethical principle of beneficence supports the advocacy role.

Advocacy becomes a central obligation when epidemiologists accept a commitment to disease prevention and control; unfortunately, this commitment is not universal.

6.7 Conclusion

If epidemiology rises to these five key challenges its healthy development in the twenty first century will be assured. If, on the other hand, it ignores the challenges, its future will be bleak, with epidemiology becoming increasingly confined to clinical epidemiology.

A flourishing discipline of epidemiology will conform to the following principles: it will be closely interconnected with the population being studied; it will be informed and guided by a theory which integrates the historical, social and economic determinants of health and disease in populations; and it will address the health problems of all groups in both the rich and poor worlds. A socially responsible epidemiology will be closely connected with public health at a global level and comprehensive solutions will emerge to confront the major health problems, rather than the current piecemeal disease by disease solutions.

Chapter 6   Key Points

The major challenges facing epidemiology are:
- to improve basic epidemiological information;
- to refine causal mechanisms and pathways and clarify the process of causal inference, focusing especially on the social origins of disease;
- to study and confront the health effects of war, poverty and global environmental change;
- to develop and strengthen the links between epidemiological findings and their application in public policy; and
- to ensure that epidemiology reaches and maintains a high ethical standard.

References

1. Gore SM. Bovine Creutzfeldt–Jakob disease? Failures of epidemiology must be remedied. *Br Med J* 1996; **312**:791–3.
2. Coleman MP, Esteve J, Damiecki P, Arslan A, Renard H. *Trends in Cancer Incidence and Mortality*. Lyon: World Health Organization International Agency for Research on Cancer, 1993.
3. WHO MONICA Project Investigators. The World Health Organization MONICA Project (monitoring trends and determinants in cardiovascular

disease: a major international collaboration. *J Clin Epidemiol* 1988; **41**:105–14.

4. Murray CJL, Lopez AL, Jamison D. The global burden of disease in 1990: summary results, sensitivity analysis and future directions. *Bull WHO* 1994; **72**:495–509.

5. Laporte RE. How to improve monitoring and forecasting of disease patterns. *Br Med J* 1993; **307**:1573–4.

6. Loomis D, Wing S. Is molecular epidemiology a germ theory for the end of the twentieth century? *Int J Epidemiol* 1990; **19**:1–3.

7. Vandenbroucke JP. Epidemiology in transition: a historical hypothesis. *Epidemiology* 1990; **1**:164–7.

8. Mosley WH, Chen LC. An analytical framework for the study of child survival in developing countries. *Pop Dev Review* 1984; **10** (Suppl.):25–45.

9. Evans RG, Stoddart GL. Producing health, consuming health care. *Soc Sci Med* 1990; **31**:1347–63.

10. Beaglehole R. Conceptual frameworks for the investigation of mortality from major cardiovascular diseases. In: Lopez A, Caselli G, Valkonen T (eds). *Adult Mortality in Developed Countries: From Description to Explanation.* Oxford: Oxford University Press, 1995.

11. Haines A, Epstein PR, McMichael AJ, on behalf of an international panel. Global health watch: monitoring impacts of environmental change. *Lancet* 1993; **342**:1464–9.

12. McMichael AJ. *Planetary Overload. Global Environmental Change and the Health of Human Species.* Cambridge: Cambridge University Press, 1993.

13. Wing S. Limits of epidemiology. *Med Global Survival* 1994; **1**:74–86.

14. Milio N. Beyond informatics: an electronic community infrastructure for public health. *J Pub Hlth Man Pract* 1995; **1**:84–94.

15. World Health Organisation Ad Hoc Committee on Health Research Relating to Future Intervention Options. *Investing in Health Research and Development* Geneva: WHO, 1996.

16. Peto R. Smoking and death: the past 40 years and the next 40. *Br Med J* 1994; **309**:937–9.

17. Rothman KJ. Policy recommendations in epidemiology research papers. *Epidemiology* 1993; **4**:94–5

18. Macdonald SC. Authors should be expected to elucidate policy implications of empirical data. *Epidemiology* 1993; **4**:557–8.

19. Rothman KJ, Poole C. Science and policy making. *Am J Pub Hlth* 1985; **75**:340–1.

20. Anon. Do epidemiologists cause epidemics? *Lancet* 1993; **341**:993–4.

21. Guidotti TL, Jacobs P. The implications of an epidemiological mistake: a community's response to a perceived excess cancer risk. *Am J Pub Hlth* 1993; **83**:233–9.

22. Fahey T, Griffiths S, Peters TJ. Evidence based purchasing: understanding results of clinical trials and systematic reviews. *Br Med J* 1995; **311**:1056–60.

23. Tabár L, Fagerberg G, Gad A, Baldetorp L Holmeberg LH, Gröntoft O, Lundström B, Månson JC. Reductions in mortality from breast cancer after mass screening with mammography. *Lancet* 1985; **i**:829–32.

24. White KL. *Healing the Schism. Epidemiology, Medicine, and the Public's Health.* New York: Springer, 1991.

25. Stolley PD. When genius errs: RA Fisher and the lung cancer controversy. *Am J Epidemiol* 1991; **133**:16–25.

26. Brown P. Popular epidemiology challenges the system. *Environment* 1993;

35:16–41.

27. Pearce N. Traditional epidemiology, modern epidemiology, and public health. *Am J Pub Hlth* 1996; **86**:678–83.

28. Susser M, Susser E. Choosing a future for epidemiology: I. Eras and paradigms. *Am J Publ Hlth*, 1996; **86**:668–73.

29. Fee E, Fox DM. *AIDS: The Burdens of History*. Berkeley: University of California Press, 1988.

30. Susser M, Susser E. Choosing a future for epidemiology: II. From black box to Chinese boxes and eco-epidemiology. *Am J Publ Hlth*, 1996; **86**:674–7.

31. World Medical Association. *Declaration of Helsinki*. Adopted by the 18th World Medical Assembly, Helsinki, Finland, June 1964, and amended by the 29th World Medical Assembly, Tokyo, Japan, October 1975; the 35th World Medical Assembly, Venice, Italy, October 1983; and the 41st World Medical Assembly, Hong Kong, September 1989.

32. Last JM. Guidelines on ethics for epidemiologists. *Int J Epidemiol* 1990; **19**:226–9.

33. Westrin C-G, Nilstun T. The ethics of data utilisation: a comparison between epdemiology and journalism. *Br Med J* 1994; **308**:522–3.

34. Anon. Protecting individuals; preserving data. *Lancet* 1992; **339**:784.

35. Lynge E. New draft on European directive on confidential data. At last, a step forward for epidemiological research. *Br Med J* 1995; **310**:1024.

36. Lynge E. European directive on confidential data: A threat to epidemiology. *Br Med J* 1994; **308**:490.

37. Barker DJP. *Fetal and Infant Orgins of Adult Disease*. London: British Medical Journal, 1992.

38. Bailar JC. Surgery for early breast cancer – can less be more? *New Engl J Med* 1995; **333**:1496–8.

39. Khan KS. Epidemiology and ethics: the perspective of the Third World. *J Pub Hlth Pol* 1994; **15**:218–25.

40. Levine C. Ethics, epidemiology, and women's health. *Ann Epidemiol* 1994; **4**:159–65.

41. Merkatz RB, Temple R, Sobel S, Feiden K, Kessler DA. Women in clinical trials of new drugs: a change in Food and Drug Administration Policy. *New Engl J Med* 1993; **329**:292–6.

42. Bankowski Z, Bryant JH, Last JM (eds). *Ethics and Epidemiology: International Guidelines*. Geneva: CIOOMS, 1991.

43. Godlee F. The Cochrane Collaboration. *Br Med J* 1994; **309**:969–70.

44. Coughlin SS, Etheredge GD. On the need for ethics curricula in epidemiology. *Epidemiology* 1995; **6**:566–7.

45. Weed DL. Science, ethics guidelines, and advocacy in epidemiology. *Ann Epidemiol* 1994; **4**:166–71.

Part III
Public health

The final part of this book considers the state of public health from both historical and contemporary perspectives. The underlying themes are the global threats to public health and the marginalisation of public health services. The prospects for major reform of public health services are assessed.

- Chapter 7 identifies recurrent themes in the history of public health which continue to influence public health practice and debates about the future of public health.
- Chapter 8 reviews the organisation and practice of public health in several wealthy countries.
- Chapter 9 examines the state of public health in selected poor countries.
- Chapter 10 assesses the prospects for public health in the new millennium.

7

Public health themes: historical and contemporary

7.1 Introduction

This chapter outlines recurrent themes in the history of public health which continue to influence public health practice and debates about the future of public health. Of central importance is the realisation that public health is not proceeding along a linear and triumphant march[1].

This chapter focuses on these themes but is not a systematic history of public health which has been covered in numerous books and articles[1-5].

7.2 The nature and scope of public health

A recurrent and critical theme concerns the nature and scope of public health. What are the boundaries of public health? How does public health relate to medical care, social welfare, environmental and occupational health? Should public health be centrally and explicitly concerned with the social and economic determinants of health, such as income, housing and poverty? The prevailing social and economic ideology has a great bearing on the answers to these questions and the emphasis given to various public health strategies. These questions are not new; the tension between a narrow medical view of public health and a broader focus on the social and economic causes of health and disease was a feature of nineteenth century public health in England[6].

Public health has been defined in many different ways. All definitions of public health have in common the idea that public health is defined in terms of its aims – to reduce disease and maintain health of the whole population – rather than by a theoretical framework or a specific body of knowledge.

In 1923 Winslow, a leading theoretician of the American public health movement during the first half of the twentieth century, proposed the following definition:

'the science and art of preventing disease, prolonging life, and promoting physical health and efficiency through organised community efforts for the sanitation of the environment, the control of community infections, the education of the individual in principles of personal hygiene, the organisation of medical and nursing service for the early diagnosis and preventive treatment of disease, and the development of the social machinery which will ensure to every individual in the community a standard of living adequate for the maintenance of health'[7].

The scope of this definition is broad, includes early diagnosis and treatment, and incorporates the underlying economic determinants of health.

Despite his broad definition, Winslow advocated the individual approach to public health and believed, for example, that the 'discovery of popular education as an instrument in preventive medicine, made by the pioneers in the tuberculosis movement, has proved almost as far reaching in its results as the discovery of the germ theory of disease thirty years before'. Winslow also noted, with approval, the increasing use of physicians for the examination of well people suggesting that control of the 'degenerative diseases requires nothing less than the systematic medical examination of presumably normal individuals'. More recently, the US Institute of Medicine defined public health as 'what we, as a society, do collectively to assure the conditions in which people can be healthy'[8]. This definition, as the Committee recognised, places a huge responsibility on America's public health agencies as it includes the provision of personal health care to the millions of people rejected by the rest of the health system. The favoured definition in the United Kingdom, and in many other countries, was proposed by the Acheson Report in 1987 as:

'the art and science of preventing disease, promoting health, and prolonging life through organised efforts of society'[9].

Resolution of the dilemma posed by varying interpretations of the scope of public health remains a priority. The continuing failure to agree on the scope of public health and, most importantly, on an appropriate set of strategies is confusing and debilitating. In our view, the Acheson definition is appropriate because it encompasses the essential elements of modern public health (Box 7.1). Public health should remain inclusive and broad in scope and strategies should be developed to achieve the broad aims. It is counter productive to espouse a broad definition and apply minimalist strategies, as has been the case for much of the last 150 years. We return to this theme in Chapter 10.

Box 7.1 The essential elements of modern public health theory and practice are:

- its emphasis on collective responsibility for health and the prime role of the state in protecting and promoting the public's health;
- a focus on whole populations;
- an emphasis on prevention, especially the population strategy for primary prevention;
- a concern for the underlying socioeconomic determinants of health and disease, as well as the more proximal risk factors;
- a multi-disciplinary basis which incorporates quantitative and qualitative methods as appropriate; and
- partnership with the populations served.

7.3 A 'Golden Age' of public health?

One of the enduring themes in public health is the idea of a past 'golden age' of public health. The origins of modern public health are usually traced back to the Victorian age in Britain, and the response to the social and health problems generated by rapid industrialisation. As Rosen has shown, however, the history of public health stretches back at least as far as the ancient Greeks and the Hippocratic School; and Sweden instituted public health measures to monitor the population and promote population growth in the early eighteenth century, well before industrialisation[10]

The birth of a systematic approach to public health at the beginning of the nineteenth century can be attributed to the development of the scientific spirit, the humanitarian ideal and the sense of 'public virtue', as well as the presumed economic value of preventing premature mortality. In both Britain and the United States of America, the public health movement was created by social reformers and included, but was not led by, medical practitioners.

Two main nineteenth century phases of public health are usually described: the environmental sanitation phase lasting from around 1840 to 1890, and the period of the scientific control of communicable disease, based on bacteriological discoveries and the germ theory, from 1890 to 1910. Winslow regarded this later phase as the 'Golden Age'. Most historians, however, date the beginning of the 'golden' age to the middle of the nineteenth century with the publication in 1842 of Chadwick's report on the sanitary conditions of the labouring class and the subsequent Public Health Act of 1848. Another suggestion is that the 'golden age' included both the second half of the nineteenth century and the first half of the twentieth century[11].

The late nineteenth century public health movement, and especially the locally administered preventive health measures which led to the reduction of the adverse health effects of industrialisation, made an important contribution to the development of public health[12]. The importance of the mid-nineteenth century 'golden age' of public health has been exaggerated as there was little real concern with the underlying social and economic determinants of disease[13]. As both professional and lay people saw disease causality in terms of precise invisible entities (disease agents), prevention policies were narrow and reductionist.

Chadwick, an ardent disciple of Bentham, the utilitarian political philosopher, was appointed as Assistant to the Royal Commission to inquire into the operation and administration of the Poor Laws, and his report revealed the ugly and dangerous conditions in which the working class lived. He believed the people's health was a matter of public concern and supported the principle that the state has responsibility for the health of the public[6]. As a result, public health was seen as a political activity with social and economic changes as its goal, and with local government having a major role to play[14]. It appears, however, Chadwick was not primarily interested in reducing disease. His major concern was tax reduction[13]. Chadwick and his colleagues were primarily interested in the miasmas or odours thought to be the cause of disease that arose from decaying organic matter, not the underlying poverty and general squalor. Filth became an important 'public enemy of community health'. Garbage removal was seen as the solution rather than alleviation of poverty.

The focus on miasma was a reflection of scientific orthodoxy, although a complex range of theories of disease causation co-existed[15]. Chadwick minimised the influence of poverty, believing that '. . . high prosperity in respect to employment and wages and abundant food have afforded to the labouring classes no exemptions from attacks of epidemic disease, which have been as frequent and as fatal in periods of commercial and manufacturing prosperity as in any others'[15]. This conclusion is more readily understandable in the context of Chadwick's starting point, which was the concern with the cost of charitable aid and the widespread Victorian belief that disease caused poverty. Environmental reforms, especially sanitary engineering, were supported in the belief that they would reduce disease and mortality and thus indirectly address the problem of poverty, without compromising individual responsibility or challenging personal liberty. The problems of commercial profit, disease prevention, environmental conditions and government action were intertwined but there was no attempt to challenge the social and political fabric of society[16,17].

The Board of Health, established by the Act of 1848, was both unpopular and short-lived because of the power of the vested interests it challenged. This situation has a parallel with the fate of the New Zealand Public Health Commission 150 years later, as discussed in Chapter 8. Following its demise, public health work passed from the Board of Health to a newly established committee of the Privy Council, where, under the direction of the Medical Officer John Simon, the foundations of a modern public health service were laid. Simon repudiated the Chadwick equation of public health with sanitary engineering and brought both medicine and science back into public health[6]. By 1870 the medical profession dominated public health in Britain and the focus had shifted from legislative action to administrative implementation[14].

From the 1870s a new profession emerged with the establishment of a national network of medical officers of health; social reformers were replaced by professional public health administrators[16]. The history of this professional group is central to the development of public health in Britain in the late nineteenth century. The failure to clarify the goals and practice of this profession undermined its influence over the political and economic development of the public health system. With the development of a national civil service, public health as a process of social reform, became diffused.

Despite their limited focus, the achievements of the sanitary reformers were impressive[12]; cholera, for example, was basically controlled by impressive feats of engineering. Chadwick was a powerful and influential person and even by modern standards his Report is an outstanding example of the use of quantitative and qualitative data to improve the public's health. By stimulating and initiating the legislative basis of public health, Chadwick did much to promote public health. Chadwick was a combination of social investigator, coalition builder, ideologue and administrator[6]. His legacy did not, in the long term, lead to a strong and vigorous public health movement; his ideas merged easily with the reductionist pressure stemming from the germ theory at the end of the nineteenth century. Chadwick and many of his colleagues were not able, or willing, to distinguish the agent of disease from the underlying causes, and when social and economic factors were identified, such as overcrowding and poor housing, the appropriate remedy (preventing poverty) was not recommended. Instead the focus was on sanitation and water supply, which although great advances in themselves, did little to lessen the impact of the underlying poverty.

An important exception to the narrow view expressed by the majority of the English sanitary reformers was provided by Virchow who identified the fundamental importance of the social origins of disease[18]. Virchow's views on the importance of social medicine are summarised in his report on an 1848 typhus epidemic in Upper Silesia. His analysis, based on only a three week visit to the region at the request of the Prussian Government, emphasised the underlying social, economic and cultural factors responsible for the epidemic. Instead of recommending a medical response, and in contrast to Chadwick, Virchow outlined a radical programme including full employment and universal education. The impact of these recommendations on the health of the people of Upper Silesia was limited because Virchow's ideas were not welcomed by the Government. Shortly after the publication of the report he was suspended from his hospital post.

With the liberalisation of Prussian politics, Virchow entered politics in 1861 and actively promoted the concept of the social origins of disease. Virchow firmly believed that a central concern of government should be the health of the people: 'a . . . sound constitution must affirm beyond any doubt the right of the individual to a healthy life'[18]. At a practical level he planned and implemented a sewerage disposal system for Berlin. Throughout his life he promoted public health against those who wanted to leave the field to private endeavour. He believed passionately that the state had to practice public health, although he was also a strong advocate for local government and decentralised interventions. Unfortunately, Virchow's ideas have not prevailed in the last 150 years.

From a historical perspective, the second half of the nineteenth century was important for public health, even if the period does not warrant the 'golden age' label. Progress was made in improving the health of the public by the sanitary reformers and their engineers. Unfortunately, the critical public health issue of poverty did not receive the attention it deserved and the sanitary reformers directed attention away from the fundamentally important social factors. From the contemporary perspective, it is still necessary for public health practitioners to focus attention on the underlying social and economic causes of health and disease. We are still awaiting the 'golden age' of public health.

7.4 Role of the state

The state has always had a major influence on public health. Usually, the state acts positively to promote health. Unfortunately, examples abound of actions taken by states that have been detrimental to health; for example, war, now more often civil than international, is one of the most harmful public health actions a state can undertake.

Since antiquity, the state has responded to public health problems by enacting laws, promulgating regulations and establishing organisations. Some of the earliest and most impressive responses were the engineering achievements of the Peruvians, Etruscans and Romans. Medieval citizen governments, like their Roman predecessors, hired labourers to clean streets, cisterns, and sewers, and remove garbage. Furthermore, they attempted to enforce the laws[19]. From the thirteenth century, Italian city states were at the forefront of sanitary endeavours, although progress was slow and public hygiene laws in 1700 strongly resembled those of 1300. Creation of public boards of health by Italian cities from about 1500 represented a major advance in public health practice. Quarantine was first used by Ragusa, the tiny Dalmatian colony of Venice, in 1377 but did not become widespread until the sixteenth century[19].

During the eighteenth century, the impetus for reform in public health moved northwards from Italian cities. Northern Europeans rejected the political basis for protecting public health and instead turned their attention to cleanliness, hospital building and information gathering. With the political assertion of health as a right of citizenship,which became common after 1800, the state was obliged to take an interest in public health[1].

Until the mid-nineteenth century, however, public health efforts were largely the work of voluntary groups or of local governments, especially in Great Britain where there was a great distrust of the central government which, in general, had little interest in public health. The public health actions of the early nineteenth century governments were usually in response to specific epidemic threats and were piecemeal and tentative actions motivated by fear, civic pride and religious zeal[16]. The first major national health law was the British Public Health Act of 1848. This Act was a landmark and foreshadowed the public health role of central governments even though it was strongly opposed by the medical profession and local government officials reluctant to surrender authority to a central agency.

In France, a system of weak local advisory health councils was established following the Revolution of 1848 and remained in effect until the end of the nineteenth century. Despite the work of the French hygienists, public health in France lagged far behind that of Britain, largely because of the lack of central government action. The public health regulations in Russia, although advanced, were not systematically enforced, even in response to cholera epidemics. In the United States of America there was a greater exertion of local control and delayed action by the federal Government.

In the twentieth century, the state became increasingly involved in public health. For example, the United States Federal Children's Bureau was established in 1912 to protect the health of children. Federal activities in public health in the United States of America gradually expanded and the Marine Hospital Service was renamed the Public Health Service in 1912. Increasing federal support was stimulated by the poor state of recruits for World Wars I and II, and in response to the economic depression of the 1930s. The federal funds were directed toward specific diseases, especially tuberculosis, and specific population groups, especially children[20].

Following the Second World War, debate occurred in the United States of America on the relationship between public health and medical care, but the federal programme for building hospitals set the agenda and diverted the bulk of federal resources into hospitals. The post-war boom in expenditure for laboratory research and hospitals was associated with the relative neglect of public health services and a failure to adopt and implement a broad view of public health[21]. By the 1970s, the financial impact of the expansion in public health activities from the 1930s, particularly the costs of medical care, began to be felt in the United States of America. As new public health issues surfaced, separate agencies were established, for example the Environmental Protection Agency. In the process, public health lost a clear institutional base and an associated loss of visibility and credibility. In the 1980s federal funding for public health programmes was cut and responsibilities shifted to the states which had the unenviable aim of tailoring limited funds to a vast array of problems.

The United States of America, along with most other countries, continues to grapple with the problems of cost escalation in health services, the emergence of new health problems, such as AIDS, and the large segment of the population without organised medical care coverage. Central to this dilemma is the argument about the scope of public health and the extent of public sector responsibility for medical care. In many countries this dilemma has been resolved by the state taking as much responsibility for individual medical care as it does for public health.

Although the state has ultimate responsibility for public health, it is often unwilling to exercise this responsibility in a planned and co-ordinated manner. Throughout history the state has been confronted by a combination of strong vested interests and a weak public health constituency and this contributes to the neglect of public health in the face of other pressing priorities. In all countries, the resources devoted by the state to public health are only a tiny fraction of those spent on medical care.

7.5 Individual liberty and collective responsibility

By definition, public health involves collective action to protect and promote health. The degree of emphasis, however, placed on collective as opposed to individual actions, has varied, often quite markedly. As a result surprisingly rapid changes have occurred in the balance of responsibilities. Collective actions have been easier to initiate, organise and implement in response to public health crises and public panic. These crises have usually involved epidemics of infectious disease, although the general health problems caused by rapid industrialisation in the eighteenth and nineteenth centuries were seen as a major threat to social order.

In the United States of America, organised public health activities began in the eighteenth century with the initiation of laws for the isolation of smallpox patients and for ship quarantine. The need for quarantine was balanced against the need to maintain trade; quarantine regulations were vigorously opposed by those whose economic investments were threatened. Prior to the twentieth century, there were few formal institutional bases for public health officials in the United States of America and, at least until the mid-nineteenth century, public health was usually the responsibility of the social elite with public health programmes being organised locally. This pattern was also common in other countries, for example Russia, where the gentry took responsibility, albeit limited, for the health of their serfs.

The recurring threat of cholera from the 1830s provided the stimulus to create boards of health in many eastern cities of the United States of America. Quarantine regulations fluctuated depending on the balance of threats from epidemics and merchants. The Civil War, in which more casualties were the result of disease than battle, emphasised the importance of infectious diseases. The industrial transformation of the north, which followed the war, exacerbated public health problems. An increasing number of reform groups took an interest in these problems and supported the need for sanitary reform. Public health reform offered a safe response to pressing social problems. In the United States of America, as elsewhere, little effort was made to tackle the underlying issue of poverty. The nineteenth century sanitarians were not afraid to tackle vested interests (water companies, landlords) but they did not oppose the underlying social and political framework. Public health had little impact on the social and economic factors crucial to the prevention of disease and the promotion of health for a number of reasons (see Box 7.2).

The main contemporary 'health crisis' in all countries is the cost of medical care stimulated by technological developments, ageing of the

---

Box 7.2   There are several reasons why public health has taken a narrow
path:

- the domination of the narrow engineering view of public health,
  stemming from Chadwick and other nineteenth century reformers, is of
  critical importance.
- the difficulty in converting a broad view of public health into appropriate
  strategies. All too often, minimalist strategies have been advocated by
  public health practitioners as a way of avoiding political conflict.
- the enormous success and popularity of the germ theory of disease
  undermined a broader public health approach at the end of the
  nineteenth century.
- the continuing lack of a public health constituency; public support for
  public health is, at best, limited. Even the limited public support is easily
  overcome by vested interests and the pressing need for governments to
  respond to immediate crises.

---

population, epidemics of non-communicable diseases, and by the need for
the medical profession to maintain its status and income[22]. Cost containment is the main motivation for health reforms in all countries, and a focus
on individual responsibility has become the main strategy for the control
and prevention of non-communicable diseases. 'Blaming the victim' (from
the 'unworthy poor' to the 'irresponsible smoker') becomes a powerful
excuse for limiting government action, a theme that has been recurrent in
public health for centuries.

The basis of effective public health strategies is collective action.
Regrettably, most government actions are a result of strong and persistent
lobbying pressure from health advocacy groups and do not stem from a
coherent approach to disease prevention and health promotion.

7.6 The role of scientific knowledge

The prevailing scientific paradigm has a strong influence on public health
practice. For centuries, the miasma theory competed with the contagion
theory of disease transmission, although these and other theories often co-
existed. The most striking impact of medical knowledge on public health
was the explosion of interest in bacteriology in the half century from 1870.
The bacteriological era overshadowed the environmental approach to
public health which had been the major strategy in the earlier decades of
the nineteenth century. By the early 1900s, bacteriology dominated the

public health agenda in both the United States of America and Europe. Once it was widely believed that it was not dirt itself that caused disease, the public health focus narrowed and attention was deflected from the primary role of the environment in disease causation.

Public health agencies began to expand their activities into laboratory science and infectious disease epidemiology. More generally, specific control measures based on laboratory sciences came to replace social and sanitary reform measures to combat disease. The focus was now on specific routes of transmission, rather than on cleaning up cities. Bacteriology became the foundation of the new scientific public health and drew attention away from the larger and more difficult problems created by poverty[23].

At the end of the twentieth century we are witnessing another paradigmatic shift with the increasing emphasis on the molecular and genetic basis of disease. The implications for public health of this shift could be profound because molecular epidemiology emphasises the technical, rather than the social and environmental, approach to disease control. Health economics has also become an important influence on public health because of the worldwide economic constraints on health spending. The World Bank has taken the initiative by identifying cost effective public health initiatives which may yield large benefits at low cost. An 'essential public health package' includes:

- childhood immunisation and micronutrient supplementation;
- school health programmes;
- public information programmes;
- programmes to reduce tobacco and alcohol consumption; and
- AIDS prevention programmes[24].

While it is, of course, important to ensure that resources are used effectively, the World Bank's approach reduces public health practice to a series of specific interventions far removed from the broad social movements which, historically, have had a greater impact on the public's health. A challenging research issue concerns the nature and origins of social movements for health and their relationship with democratic traditions. Some insights into this issue can be gained from countries that have achieved an exceptional health status at relatively low cost, as will be discussed in Chapter 9.

7.7 The professionalisation of public health

The professionalisation of public health is now linked to the development of specialised knowledge in medicine. The history of public health in early nineteenth century Europe and the United States of America is replete with reformers, many of whom were not health professionals; the role of doctors was limited in the Victorian public health efforts. All reforms were motivated by the notion that ill health caused poverty which, in turn, led to unproductive expenditure on poor relief and further demoralisation of the poor.

Public health programmes in the nineteenth century were promoted by a variety of interest groups for many different reasons. Some were directly concerned about health on humanitarian or religious grounds. Others saw health as a social issue central to the stability of the state. Nineteenth century public health adopted a healthy public policy approach only in so far as central and local governments were involved in episodic attempts to regulate against public health dangers and to implement sanitary reform. The early public health reformers, often described as 'zealots', were strongminded and dedicated people[16]. Unfortunately, the concept of public health remained indistinct and was characterised by the absence of a coherent philosophy. Despite the professionalisation of public health, this criticism remains valid today.

The public health movement in the United Kingdom embraced medical practitioners only towards the end of the nineteenth century. The first medical officer of health was appointed in Liverpool in 1847[25]. The professionalisation of public health in Great Britain continued with the Public Health Act of 1872 which made the appointment of a medical officer of health obligatory for local sanitary authorities. Medical officers of health were responsible for enforcing public health acts in their communities, for inspecting food, sanitation and housing, and for publishing an annual report on their activities and the state of public health in their communities.

In the early years of the twentieth century there was a narrowing of focus towards the responsibility of the individual for 'personal prevention', with health education as the main strategy. Medical officers of health in the United Kingdom also became involved in hospital administration, although this responsibility was removed with the formation of the National Health Service in 1948[4]. At the same time, public health moved closer to clinical medicine despite the desire of some academic social medicine advocates and political lobby groups to broaden the focus of public health. As public health became a 'special kind of clinical medicine', practical public health was neglected, especially in the 1930s when medical officers of health became responsible for administering clinical services and hospitals. Social medicine, which espoused a broad view of public health, remained confined to universities. Social medicine was quite separate from health policy and practical public health[26] and contributed to the rift between public health teaching and practice.

In the United States of America the medicalisation of public health occurred later, beginning in the 1920s. Until this time it was largely the field of engineers, biologists and a few social scientists[27]. The key event in this process was the establishment in 1916 of the Johns Hopkins School of Hygiene and Public Health with the financial support of the Rockefeller Foundation.

In the United Kingdom, the speciality of Community Medicine was established in the early 1970s as the 'speciality practised by epidemiologists and administrators of medical services'[16]. This speciality became embedded within the structure of the health service and was not able, or willing, to articulate a concern for a broad vision of public health. A few notable public health academics, such as Cochrane, were willing to question the value of medical care activities[28]. In general, the difficult task of addressing the underlying causes of ill health was not given priority by the public health professions. To its credit, the Community Medicine speciality has, at times, argued for a social view of public health, for example, in response to the Black Report on inequalities[29].

The speciality of public health has continued to evolve. In many countries, such as the United Kingdom, Australia and New Zealand, it is strongly influenced by the medical profession. In the United States of America, public health has a much broader constituency and the medical profession is not dominant. A broad and inclusive public health speciality is the only viable option in countries where public health specialists of all disciplinary backgrounds are rare. One possible outcome of a broad based disciplinary grouping is the lowering of status of public health professionals, in comparison with the medical profession. This is a small price to pay, however, as the medicalisation of public health has itself resulted in a narrowing of the focus of public health practice. The Faculty of Public Health Medicine (the modern form of the specialty of Community Medicine) has explored ways of opening its membership to non-medically qualified public health practitioners. Unfortunately the Faculty has been unable to achieve internal consensus on this proposal with the opposition coming largely from younger members who feel that their career prospects would be damaged by the ending of the medical monopoly on senior public health posts[30].

An unresolved issue for medically qualified public health practitioners is their relationship with clinical medicine[26]. In the United Kingdom, Australia and New Zealand, public health medicine has emerged as a distinct entity on the basis of clinical epidemiology and 'evidence-based medicine'. While this development is good for clinical medicine and increases the status of public health medicine, it is a diversion from the main challenges facing public health. It is unlikely that this development will, in itself, renew public health. In the medium term, it would be more product- ive for public health doctors to return to the mainstream of public health and to resist co-option and integration with clinical medicine[31].

7.8 Internationalisation of public health

Victorian England influenced the development of public health in North America, although, largely because of the size of the continent, there was a greater tendency for decentralised activity at the state level. The impact of the Victorian approach to health and welfare was felt most directly on the English colonies, especially in India[32], Africa and Australasia[33]. As we will see in Chapter 9, this influence continues today. Other colonial powers had a similar and longstanding impact on the practice of public health in their colonies. This influence is not new; the Hippocratic writings on the effects of the environment provided useful advice for the colonisation of ancient Greece[1].

The experience of the United States Army in the Spanish–American War in Cuba and the Philippines with yellow fever and malaria illustrates the importance of public health for successful colonisation[34]. These lessons were applied in the southern United States of America with the support of Rockefeller money. By 1915 the Public Health Service, the United States Army and the Rockefeller Foundation were the major agencies involved in public health in the United States and its colonies.

The modern form of colonialism is less direct, but equally influential. Many international agencies, including the World Bank and the International Monetary Fund, play an important part in shaping eco- nomic, welfare and health policies in poor countries. Recent structural adjustment programmes, put in place to facilitate debt repayment, have encouraged the move towards market based approaches to medical care and public health policy. The health impact of these programmes has yet to be comprehensively described, although it appears that the health problems of many people in poor countries have been exacerbated. We return to this theme in Chapter 9.

A feature of international public health has been the attempts to eradi- cate selected diseases. This concept probably originated with the Rockefeller Foundation at its inception in 1913[35]. Eradication of hookworm was the major goal, although the technology was not, and is still not, available for this task. Yellow fever and malaria eradication programmes followed in 1955, both of which were only partially successful; there has been a massive resurgence in malaria since the successes of the 1950s and 1960s. It is now appreciated that the discipline of tropical medicine achieved more for the health of the colonialists than for tropical countries[36].

The eradication of smallpox was successful with the last naturally occurring case being found in Somalia in 1977 after a ten year campaign led by WHO. Despite this success, there was a general disillusionment with disease targeted approaches. The Alma Ata Declaration of 1978 encapsulated the comprehensive primary health care approach defined as 'essential health care made universally accessible to individuals and families in the community by means acceptable to them, through their full participation and at a cost that the community and country can afford'[37]. The overall goal endorsed by WHO was the 'attainment by all peoples of the world by the year 2000 of a level of health that will permit them to lead a socially and economically productive life'. Fine words, but the year 2000 is close and the rhetoric has not matched the achievements. In part, the recession of the 1980s is to blame. The resources made available, however, did not match the policy goals and where resources were available, they were not necessarily directed to public health policy goals.

In the 1980s the international goal of comprehensive primary health care was replaced by 'selective primary health care' which targets, in the interim, the few most important diseases for which cost effective therapies are available (Box 7.3). Four key interventions were developed and implemented: immunisation, oral rehydration, breast feeding, and antimalarial drugs. In 1983, UNICEF spearheaded this initiative with the goal of universal childhood immunisation.

7.9 Conclusion

The challenges facing public health at the end of the twentieth century are not new. All current challenges have historical antecedents and lessons abound as we approach the twenty first century. Unfortunately, the situation confronting public health practitioners is now especially difficult. The globalisation of trade, the dependence of poor countries on a few wealthy countries for aid, the integration of labour markets in poor countries with the needs of multinational companies, all increase the difficulty of dealing with public health issues at a country level. A central challenge is to develop a global approach to public health: a challenge we return to in Chapter 10.

Box 7.3 Differing approaches to health care

Comprehensive primary health care and selective primary health care are fundamentally different approaches[38].

- Primary health care is based on the broad definition of health; selective primary health care views health as the absence of disease.
- Primary health care stresses equity; selective primary health care consolidates the power of health professionals and promotes technological solutions to health problems. Selective primary health care has been particularly directed towards improving child health, although the 1993 World Development Report expands this approach to adults.
- Comprehensive primary health care stresses the necessity of multisector approaches to health; selective primary health care focuses on the prevention and management of selected important disease problems.
- Primary health care is firmly rooted in community empowerment; with selective primary health care, community involvement is necessary only for compliance, not for decision making and control. Comprehensive primary health care is an essential component of broad and inclusive public health practice.

Chapter 7 Key Points

The recurrent historical themes that continue to influence public health practice are:
- the lack of agreement on the scope of public health and the appropriate strategies;
- the belief in a 'golden age' of public health;
- the central but varying role of the state;
- the tension between individual liberty and collective responsibility;
- the influence of scientific knowledge on public health practice;
- the professionalisation of public health; and
- the internationalisation of public health.

References

1. Porter D (ed.). *The History of Public Health and the Modern State*. Amsterdam: Editions Rodopi BV, 1994.
2. Rosen G. *From Medical Police to Social Medicine: Essays on the History of Health Care*. New York: Science History Publications, 1974.
3. Duffy J. *The Sanitarians. A History of American Public Health*. Chicago: University of Illinois Press, 1990.

4. Lewis J. The origins and development of public health in the UK. In: Holland WW, Detels R, Knox G (eds). *Oxford Textbook of Public Health: Influences of Public Health.* Oxford: Oxford University Press, 1991.
5. Lewis J. The public's health: philosophy and practice in Britain in the twentieth century. In: Fee E, Acheson R (eds). *A History of Education in Public Health. Health that Mocks the Doctors' Rules.* Oxford: Oxford University Press, 1991.
6. Hamlin C. State medicine in Great Britain. In: Porter D (ed.) *The History of Public Health and the Modern State.* Amsterdam: Editions Rodopi BV, 1994.
7. Winslow CEA. *The Evolution and Significance of the Modern Public Health Campaign.* New York: Yale University Press, 1923.
8. Committee for the Study of the Future of Public Health. *The Future of Public Health.* Washington: National Academy Press, 1988.
9. Committee of Inquiry into the Future Development of the Public Health Function. *Public Health In England.* London: HMSO, Cmd 289, 1988.
10. Johannisson K. The people's health: public health policies in Sweden. In: Porter D (ed.). *The History of Public Health and the Modern State.* Amsterdam: Editions Rodopi BV, 1994.
11. Nijhuis HGJ, Van Der Maesen LJG. The philosophical foundations of public health: an invitation to debate. *J Epidemiol Comm Hlth* 1994; **48**:1–3.
12. Szreter S. The importance of social intervention in Britain's mortality decline c.1850–1914: a re-interpretation of the role of public health. *Soc Social Hist Med* 1988; **1**:1–37.
13. Tesh SN. Miasma and 'social factors' in disease causality: lessons from the nineteenth century. *J Hlth Pol Pol Law* 1996; **20**:1001–31.
14. Fee E, Porter D. Public health, preventive medicine and professionalization: England and America in the nineteenth century. In: Wear A (ed.). *Medicine in Society.* Cambridge: Cambridge University Press, 1992.
15. Pelling M. *Cholera, Fever and English Medicine 1825–1865.* Oxford: Oxford University Press, 1978.
16. Lewis J. *What Price Community Medicine? The Philosophy, Practice and Politics of Public Health since 1919.* Sussex: Wheatsheaf Books, 1986.
17. Ringen K. Chadwick, the maket ideology, and sanitary reform: on the nature of the 19th-century public health movement. *Int J Hlth Serv* 1979; **9**:107–20.
18. Taylor R, Rieger A. Medicine as social science: Rudolf Virchow on the typhus epidemic in Upper Silesia. *Int J Hlth Serv* 1985; **15**:547–59.
19. Carmichael AG. History of public health and sanitation in the west before 1700. In: Kiple KF (ed.). *The Cambridge World History of Human Disease.* Cambridge: Cambridge University Press, 1993.
20. Snyder LP. Passage and significance of the 1944 Public Health Service Act. *Pub Hlth Reports* 1994; **109**:721–4.
21. Fox DM. The Public Health Service and the Nation's health care in the post-World War II era. *Pub Hlth Reports* 1994; **109**:725–7.
22. Evans RG, Stoddart GL. Producing health, consuming health care. *Soc Sci Med* 1990; **31**:1347–63.
23. Hill HW. *The New Public Health.* New York: Macmillan, 1916.
24. World Development Report, 1993. *Investing in Health, World Development Indicators.* New York: Oxford University Press, 1993.
25. Porter D. Stratification and its discontents: professionalization and conflict in the British Public Health Service, 1848–1914. In: Fee E, Acheson R (eds). *A History of Education in Public Health. Health that Mocks the Doctors' Rules.* Oxford: Oxford University Press, 1991.

26. Holland WW, Fitzsimons B, O'Brien M. 'Back to the future' – public health research into the next century. *J Pub Hlth Med* 1994; **16**:4–10.
27. Acheson RM. The medicalization of public health; the United Kingdom and the United States contrasted. *J Pub Hth Med* 1990; **12**:31–8.
28. Cochrane A. *Effectiveness and Efficiency*. London: Nuffield Provinical Hospitals Trust, 1972.
29. Smith A, Jacobson B. *The Nation's Health: A Strategy for the 1990s.* London: King Edward's Hospital Fund, 1988.
30. Scally G. Public health medicine in a new era. *Soc Sci Med* 1996; **42**:777–80.
31. Leeder SR. Improving our self-episteme. *Aust J Pub Hlth* 1994; **18**:355.
32. Harrison M. *Public Health in British India: Anglo-Indian Preventive Medicine 1859–1914*. Cambridge: Cambridge University Press, 1994.
33. Maclean FS. *Challenge for Health. A History of Public Health in New Zealand*. Wellington: Government Printer, 1964.
34. Fee E. Public health and the state: the United States. In: Porter D (ed.). *The History of Public Health and the Modern State*. Amsterdam: Editions Rodopi BV, 1994.
35. Warren KS. Tropical medicine or tropical health: the Heath Clark Lectures, 1988. *Rev Infect Dis* 1990; **12**:142–56.
36. Ramirez VD. Will tropical medicine move to the tropics? *Lancet* 1996; **347**:629–31.
37. World Health Organization. *Alma-Ata. Primary Health Care (Health For All Series No.1)*. Geneva: World Health Organization, 1978.
38. Rifkin SB, Walt G. Why health improves: defining the issues concerning 'comprehensive primary health care' and 'selective primary health care'. *Soc Sci Med* 1986; **6**:559–66.

8

Public health organisation and practice in wealthy countries

8.1 Introduction

This chapter assesses the current state of public health in five wealthy countries: the United Kingdom, United States of America, Sweden, Japan and New Zealand. The United Kingdom is included because of its historical importance for the development of modern epidemiology and public health. The United States is important because of its wealth and the dominance of the private sector in the provision of health care. Sweden, by contrast, has a stronger commitment to public welfare. Japan has undergone remarkable improvements in health standards over the last half century and it is of interest to see whether public health reforms have been a key to these changes. New Zealand, although a tiny country by world standards, has had a long commitment to public welfare and recent major changes to the organisation and delivery of health care led, briefly, to an unusual institutional rearrangement of public health.

An obvious gap is a country from Central and Eastern Europe. As the rate of change is so rapid in most of these countries and information scarce, it was not appropriate to include one of these countries; the developing role of the European Union in health affairs is described. It is also apparent that some countries which have made major gains in public health recently, such as The Netherlands, have been omitted, as have states which have achieved more than the country as a whole, for example, Victoria in Australia[1]. The situation in selected poorer countries will be described in the next chapter.

There have been several international comparisons of national health systems, although all focus on the organisation and delivery of personal medical care services[2]. In contrast, there have been few comparable studies focusing on public health systems[3]. From a research perspective, it would be desirable to assess all aspects of national public health institutions and organisations, including central and local governmental and non-governmental organisations, the capacity of the entire public health work-force and the priority given to public health policies. With this information it would be possible to categorise national public health systems and relate these to measures of health status of populations, for example avoidable mortality[4]. Unfortunately, the data required for such a formal assessment are not available and the methods used in this survey are mostly descriptive.

8.2 Public health in the United Kingdom

The United Kingdom, as the first industrial nation, was the first to respond to the major public health problems caused by industrialisation and urban-isation, and for a brief period in the mid-nineteenth century, there was a close relationship between epidemiology and public health. In this century many of the major developments in epidemiology have been instituted in the United Kingdom, including the studies on tobacco and disease by Doll and Hill, medical record linkage studies, mega-trials, clinical epidemiology, and the Cochrane Collaboration. Furthermore, many important intellec-tual contributions to epidemiology and public health have come from United Kingdom scientists[5]. The academic epidemiology journals pub-lished in the United Kingdom have maintained a closer connection with public health than the journals from the United States of America.

Although the United Kingdom public health experience has been a model for other countries, much has been unique to the United Kingdom; many developments differ within the United Kingdom, sometimes on a town-to-town basis[6]. Furthermore, recent national developments have exposed the fragility of the public health services following deregulation, the Conservative Government's main strategy for health reform. As a con-sequence, there has been little effective broad public health action in the United Kingdom over recent decades. The crisis over Creutzfeldt–Jakob disease is the latest illustration of the adverse effect on public health of the abrogation of government responsibility[7].

The health services, including public health services, have been reorgan-ised repeatedly over the last two decades. The status of public health doctors in the twentieth century, especially in urban areas, has been low, in contrast to their high status in the second half of the nineteenth century. A major feature of the recent history of public health has been the struggle to improve their status, at the expense of the broad specialty of public health.

Following the foundation of the National Health Service in 1948, public health in the 1950s and 1960s drifted without a strong identity, but with an increasing concern with the provision of personal preventive services[8]. A split developed between academic social medicine and practical public health in the United Kingdom[8,9], although some professors of public health were also district public health officers or medical officers of health. In this period academic public health, and especially epidemiology, flourished. In contrast, the practical side of public health declined.

The new speciality of Community Medicine was created in the mid-1970s based on the recommendations of a Royal Commission on Medical Education which suggested the amalgamation of academic social medicine and public health medicine[10]. The new speciality continued to experience the twin tensions of its relationship with the state on the one hand, and to the rest of the medical profession on the other. Unfortunately, the public health function was also removed from local authorities, thus precluding a focus on wider public health issues. The role of the medical officer of health was replaced by the 'community medicine physician'; and the requirement for annual reports on the state of public health fell into abeyance[11]. Community medicine became increasingly managerial in focus with an emphasis on the effectiveness and efficiency of personal medical services. The broad mandate of public health was forgotten in order to avoid political conflict.

The identity of community medicine was closely connected with the structure of the National Health Service and by the early 1980s the position of community medicine was undermined following National Health Service reorganisations. The 1988 Report of the Committee of Inquiry into the Future Development of the Public Health Function (the Acheson Report) advocated a return of community medicine back to 'public health medicine'[12]. The Report made a detailed set of proposals for the public health function, most of which have been adopted by the Government including the establishment of several new schools and institutes of public health, despite the paucity of staff available to fill academic vacancies[13]. Some were extensions of previous academic departments and others were extensions of service departments with little academic content.

The Report also concluded that the public health role of local health authorities should be made explicit. Regional and district health authorities were given legal responsibility for reviewing the health of the population, setting policy aims and objectives, and evaluating progress. Responsibility was also given to local health authorities to control communicable disease outbreaks. An important aspect of the post-Acheson public health function was the production of annual reports for National Health Service districts and regions. These reports were designed to be a central component of the strategic planning and contracting process with the Health of the Nation document as the guiding plan. There remains a tension between the independence of the annual reports and corporate ownership; after all, the annual reports are written by a member of the health authority. The standard of the reports varies greatly from one area to another, their aims are not explicit, and they have not been formally evaluated.

According to Acheson, the fundamental role of public health specialists should be to give advice and monitor progress towards specified goals. This would include lobbying on policy issues, co-ordinating local intersectoral issues, and organising disease prevention services such as immunisation and screening. Despite the emphasis on prevention and health promotion, the curriculum the Report proposes gives a central place to the analysis of health service needs; the need for research is only briefly mentioned. The increase in the status of public health medicine in the last decade is due more to the indirect impact of health service reforms than to the implementation of the Acheson Report.

The major health service reorganisation in 1989 introduced the internal market to the National Health Service. Health authorities, instead of being given an arbitrary allocation by government to run their services, are allocated a budget based on the population served and are expected to buy services from the most appropriate source, the so called 'purchaser-provider split'. These reforms were welcomed by some public health physicians, although not the Faculty of Public Health Medicine, in contrast to the initial negative reaction of the rest of the medical profession[14]. On balance, the changes seemed to enhance the voice of public health medicine, although there is a danger that a preoccupation with hospital services will be at the expense of prevention and health promotion[15]. Another negative effect of the purchaser–provider split was that public health departments had to give up their provider functions in order to avoid potential conflict of interest.

Many public health physicians believe that the purchaser-provider split is in accord with the Acheson report recommendations[16]. It appears that assessment of the health of the population is focusing on health care needs, and promoting health is becoming equated with 'purchasing for health gains', a process which down plays the role of the social and economic determinants of health. Directors of public health are increasingly involved in the organisation of clinical services, to the detriment of broader public health activities; a similar trend occurred earlier in the century with the medical officers of health. Although the assessment of health care needs will not improve the public's health, it will contribute to the relief of suffering and diminution of morbidity provided by individual health care services. In theory, the purchasing function could allow public health physicians to refocus spending priorities towards effective and efficient services. In practice, there is a danger that this function could hinder collaboration among health care professionals[17]. The important public health function, to promote and maintain the health of the nation, cannot be achieved through purchasing alone because the major determinants of health lie outside the health services; public health medicine must continue to focus attention on these social, economic and political issues.

The Government's Health of the Nation document, published in 1992, set out a strategy for improving health, and included for the first time health goals and targets in several key areas. The criteria used for selecting key areas were that they should be a major cause of death or avoidable ill health; that cost-effective interventions were available; and setting targets and monitoring progress were possible. Although most commentators welcomed the target-setting process, the report was criticised for its failure to grapple with the social origins of ill health, and its lack of attention to health inequalities[18].

A major limitation of the government's strategy has been its unwillingness to support local action with appropriate national action, such as legislation to restrict tobacco advertising, or to provide major extra resources for public health programmes. For example, funding for the Health Education Authority for England was radically reduced in 1994 and it now has to make up the short fall by bidding for contracts. Furthermore, there have been several recent examples where the independence of the public health advice the government received has been called into question[19].

Another report on public health medicine in the United Kingdom appeared in 1993, the Abrams Report[20], stimulated by the 'urgent need to clarify the public health function' following the changes to the National Health Service since the Acheson Report. According to this Report, all parts of the National Health Service were expected to work to improve the nation's health and directors of public health were charged with providing a comprehensive district public health strategy which closely integrates the work of general practitioners, local government and other health care providers. Unfortunately, disputes over professional boundaries have not been resolved by this Report. Of greater concern is that the Abrams Report focused only on the medical contribution to public health and ignored the more important social and economic determinants of health. There is a danger that public health physicians will again be encouraged to emphasize their management role at the expense of advisory and advocacy functions. The ongoing tensions between public and political accountability and professional autonomy have yet to be resolved. At the same time, public health resources are being cut to reduce the so called 'management costs' of purchasing[21]. A worrying aspect of these new developments has been the takeover by purchase and contracting directors of the health strategy, previously the responsibility of the directors of public health.

The latest development in the National Health Service, and one which is on the agenda in other countries, is for 'primary care led purchasing'. This is a continuation of general practice fund holding in which general practitioners are given responsibility for administering budgets provided by the district health authority. Although this development will no doubt improve specific public health programmes, for example cervical screening, it will inevitably lead to further fragmentation of health services and reduced opportunities for planning on a population-wide basis. A potential result of this development is that the purchasing process will relate more to the needs of the individual patients than to the needs of populations[22]. While it may be possible for general practitioners to develop a broader public health perspective, historically this has proved difficult[23].

In 1996, with legislation to abolish regional health authorities, the regional directors of public health and their staff became civil servants and will be even more constrained in their ability to speak out on matters of public health importance[24]. Regional directors of public health will no longer be able to publish independent annual reports, but will contribute to the report of the Chief Medical Officer.

In summary, public health in the United Kingdom remains medically dominated. Over the last two decades repeated reorganisations have hindered the development of a strong and cohesive approach to public health. The basic sciences of public health are strong, especially epidemiology and biostatistics, but much of the academic public health workforce is concentrated in only a few institutions. In contrast to the earlier decades of the National Health Service, the status of academic public health has diminished as the service role of public health has become dominant. Little effort has been devoted to developing a multi-disciplinary and intersectoral approach to health improvement in the United Kingdom. Research funding for universities is increasingly dependent on the formal assessment of the quality and quantity of publications; this exercise will make interdepartmental and multi-disciplinary collaboration more difficult. The public health workforce is fragmented and there is little sense of a co-operative movement in which a range of professionals jointly approach the tasks of researching and promoting the health of defined populations. Public health physicians increasingly concentrate on guiding the process of purchasing health services. They are also the only group with protected funding for training; financial support is required for funding the education and training of other public health professionals and for encouraging research to improve the effectiveness of public health interventions.

The outlook for public health in the United Kingdom, after over a decade of Conservative government and many reforms to the health service, is not encouraging. A major public health challenge is the increasing health inequalities in the United Kingdom[25]. There is no suggestion that public health is now a means for transforming society[6,26]. The focus remains on the role of the market in the provision of services and on the management of personal health services. This is a result of deliberate government policies which have also led to a mismatch between political solutions and public health reality. While this focus remains, health inequalities in the United Kingdom will continue to increase and preventable causes of death, disease and disability will not receive the attention they deserve. The general election in 1997 returned a government more sympathetic to public health. The Labour Party's policy on health contained in the draft election manifesto released in mid-1995 concentrated on personal health care services[27], although a senior minister for public health and a dedicated public health unit in the Department of Health are two of the ways that the Labour Government raised the profile of the discipline[28]. Rejuvenation of public health in the United Kingdom will require more than a new government; concerted effort is required to build strong coalitions of all public health professsionals and a broad public constituency.

8.3 Public health in Europe

Two agencies, the World Health Organization and the European Union, are actively engaged in setting public health policy in Europe. The World Health Organization developed a coherent and comprehensive set of 38 health targets[29]. The first major evaluation of progress in implementing the regional targets was completed in 1985 and the second in 1993. In general, progress towards better health was good and moderate progress was made towards the 'lifestyle' and environment targets. The goal of equity, however, remains elusive. The widening gap in health status between the northern/western and the central/eastern parts of Europe, with southern Europe intermediate in most respects, means that many of the health targets for Europe cannot be achieved for the region as a whole[30].

In the late 1980s a process of rapid political change began in the countries of Central and Eastern Europe, with an increasing emphasis on market forces as a guiding economic principle. The ramifications of the dissolution of the Soviet Union continue to influence the health of many Europeans[31]. The deterioration of health status in the former Soviet Union is the result of systemic social and economic breakdown consequent on its 'defeat' in the long 'cold war'. The health crisis is unlikely to be resolved until a viable political, economic, and social order is established[32].

Most national economies in the region face serious social, economic and political problems and unemployment levels are rising rapidly. By the end of the 1980s, all countries in Central and Eastern Europe for which data were available, except Poland, showed a slow down in economic growth. Differences in wealth widened, with the rich countries, regions and social groups becoming richer, and the poor relatively poorer.

Striking variations remain in death rates across the continent, and in many countries of Central and Eastern Europe life expectancy at birth declined in the 1980s, especially in men, at a time when it increased by 2.5 years in Western Europe[33]. The main contribution to the continuing high all cause mortality rates in Central and Eastern Europe since 1970, is the lack of improvement in causes of death not amenable to medical treatment, especially the preventable non-communicable diseases of adults[34]; cardiovascular disease mortality rates, for example in Central and Eastern Europe are now the highest in the world.

A detailed analysis of changes in life expectancy at birth in the 1980s in Czechoslovakia, Hungary and Poland showed that improvements in infant mortality have been counteracted by deteriorating death rates among young and middle-aged people, with the deterioration commencing as young as late childhood in Hungary but in the thirties and forties in former Czechoslovakia and Poland. The leading contributors to this deterioration are cancer and cardiovascular diseases. In Hungary, cirrhosis and accidents have also been of great importance, indicating the adverse effect of excessive alcohol consumption[33].

The practice of public health has been weak and poorly co-ordinated in Central and Eastern Europe. The first formal school of public health in Poland, established in 1991, reflects a modest resurgence in public health training in Central and Eastern Europe. In many of these countries, public health has taken a prime responsibility for managing the health system[35] and curricula in the new school of public health emphasise health service management[36]. While the latter is a major challenge, given the poor state of the health service in much of Central and Eastern Europe, it will distract from the wider goals of public health.

Opportunities abound for co-operative international public health efforts to assist the development of public health in Central and Eastern Europe[37]. A priority is the development of a critical mass of trained and experienced public health teachers[38]. Excellent examples of international cooperation in public health training exist, for example in Hungary where the new programme in public health medicine gives emphasis to non-communicable disease epidemiology and subjects such as health economics and health promotion have been introduced for the first time[39,40]. It is important that all new ventures are driven by public health needs, not commercial interests or public health 'entrepreneurs'.

Germany was a pioneer in some aspects of nineteenth century public health, for example the work of Virchow. Following the rise of Hitler, however, positive public health developments came to an end and were not reinstituted post-war. Disease prevention is now largely based on health education and there is an aversion to state supported disease control programmes[36]. Considerable local and regional variation has continued to characterise public health in Germany and there has been little integration of scientific approaches with public health programmes[41]. Public health training, administration and career structures are also not well developed in Germany and although new postgraduate training initiatives are underway[42], it is unlikely that Germany will provide strong leadership for public health in Europe in the near future.

Paradoxically France, which was also a pioneer in the early nineteenth century public hygiene movement, was slow to implement public health measures on a wide scale. Furthermore, the central government has long played a limited role in public health in France[43]. A formal public health training programme has begun in France but it is unlikely, given the weakness of public health in France, that it will provide strong leadership for the rest of Europe.

The European Union has a formal interest in public health under Article 129 of the Maastricht Treaty[44]. European Union action in public health has been limited to research, and health information and education concerning, in particular, major non-communicable diseases and drug dependence[45], but its focus is now expanding[46]. Unfortunately, the European Union health policies are fragmented and are often the indirect result of economic policies. The Commission of the European Communities published its Framework for Action in the Field of Public Health in 1993[47] and a proposal for a five-year public health programme was produced in 1995.

The plan immediately ran into strong opposition because of the contradiction between the desire of the Commission to promote health while involved in huge subsidies to the tobacco and alcohol industries[48,49]. Vested interests within Europe will probably reduce the impact of the Commission's first venture into public health. The European Union policies, to the extent that they are part of a directive, can be enforced, whereas the implementation of WHO policies is voluntary. There is scope for co-ordinated action by WHO and the European Union on public health strategies, especially in Central and Eastern Europe. The BIOMED programmes of the European Union offer some promise for the development of public health research in Europe.

A positive development for public health in Europe are the organisations that have been formed to provide leadership such as the various European groupings of epidemiologists, the European Association for Public Health, the European Alliance for Public Health, and the Association of Schools of Public Health in the European Region which is developing standard accredited public health courses and attempting to co-ordinate the development of new schools of public health[36]. It is clear that a major influence on health in Central and Eastern Europe for years to come will be the upheavals consequent upon the breakdown of the Soviet Union and its sphere of influence and the uncritical adoption of the market ideology[50].

8.4 Public health in the United States of America

The United States of America epitomises the problems wealthy countries experience when public health is neglected. The major dilemma facing public health in the United States continues to be its relationship with the organisation and delivery of medical care services. Until a national and equitable system of medical care is achieved, public health will be neglected and receive an inadequate share of the vast resources devoted to 'health' in the United States. The tremendous amount spent on medical care limits the availability of funds for a whole range of public services, not just public health.

8.4.1 Organisation of public health services

The organisation of public health in the United States of America shows huge variations among the States[51] reflecting the wide range of governmental (state, local and federal) agencies providing services. Services are also provided at national, state and local levels by environmental, occupational safety, mental health, disability, and social service groups. This fragmentation, together with a weak centralised authority, leads to great difficulty in the implementation of effective public health programmes. Public health departments have become last resort providers for uninsured patients and for patients rejected by private practitioners. Almost three-quarters of all state and local health departments expenditures are for personal health services[52]. Public health has been increasingly starved of funds and this trend has been exacerbated by the increasing use of federal block grants to states[53,54].

Although the states have primary responsibility for public health in the United States of America, the Federal Government plays a major role in defining health objectives for the nation, providing financial and technical support in achieving these objectives, and co-ordinating the efforts of the states[55]. The primary responsibility for public health at the federal level rests with the Department of Health and Human Services, with the Public Health Service, one component of the Department, having the central responsibility, although many public health activities are scattered throughout the federal bureaucracy. Within the Public Health Service, the Centers for Disease Control and the Health Resources and Services Administration are the most important public health agencies. Each state has a health agency, although some are components of larger agencies which also include social welfare and income maintenance services. The vast majority of the funds for public health services come from governmental sources, most from federal agencies.

The state health agency is headed by a state health officer appointed by the Governor in the majority of states. Most state health officers are medically qualified; increasingly these positions are political appointments. At the local government level, there are approximately 3000 local health departments serving either a single municipality or county or a group of counties. The relationship between the local health departments and local government and state health agencies are variable; some local health departments are district offices of the state health agency, some are autonomous, and some are responsible to both local government and the state health agency. Local health departments are usually responsible for the direct delivery of public health services including non-communicable disease control programmes, and maternal and child health services. A variety of restrictions imposed on local health departments, however, have considerably weakened their role in public health in the 1960s and 1970s. A recent survey of local health departments found that only 11% of 2263 departments had direct access to a trained epidemiologist or statistician on their staff [56].

The United States of America has been at the forefront of the process of setting objectives for public health, although antecedents can be found in the Canadian Lalonde Report of 1974[57]. In 1980 several initiatives culminated in a set of quantified goals for 1990 which was followed by a midcourse review in 1985[58]. While broad national goals provided a basis for accountability, no detailed action plans were provided. The overemphasis on individual responsibility and a downplaying of governmental responsibility for health were other limitations. Some progress has been made towards many of these goals, for example smoking reduction by adults, and a revised set of objectives were established for the year 2000. Many of these goals specifically address the need to reduce social and ethnic inequalities in health, although progress has been disappointingly slow in these areas[58].

8.4.2 The Institute of Medicine's Report

A committee was established by the Institute of Medicine to review the state of public health in the United States of America in the 1980s because of the perception that the nation had lost sight of its public health goals and allowed the system of public health activities to fall into disarray[59]. After a two year study, the Committee 'viewed with alarm' the state of public health. A range of problems were found: disorganisation, weak and unstable leadership, a lessening of professional public health competence, hostility to public health concepts, outdated statutes, inadequate financial support for public health activities, gaps in data gathering and surveillance, and lack of intersectoral links. The 'core' functions of public health received less than 1% of the health budget[60]. In the Committee's view, these problems reflected a lack of appreciation among the public, the policy makers and the medical profession of the central role of public health in maintaining and improving the health of the public.

The Committee was critical of short-term solutions because they too often led to fragmentation, organisational confusion, and public disenchantment; in the Committee's word – 'disarray'. Several reasons explain the disarray. Relative success in dealing with many infectious diseases led to the perception that the major public health problems were solved and there was no further need for organised public health involvement. This belief also led to a unidimensional approach to complex public health problems and encouraged the fragmentation of public health programmes among many agencies.

The Report attempted to convey an urgent message to the American public: public health is a vital function which requires broad public support in order to fulfil society's interest in assuring the conditions in which people can be healthy. The Committee recognised that restoring an effective public health system cannot be achieved by public health professionals alone. The Institute of Medicine's recommendations would have meant substantial additional resources available for public health, an integration of mental health services into health departments, and an even greater role in the provision of medical services to the poor. Similar conclusions were reached eleven years earlier, after a survey of local public health departments and their directors[61].

The Institute of Medicine's report received a mixed response. Some questioned the assumption that public health alone can fill the stated mission. Several commentators believed that the Report was unfairly negative towards public health personnel[62] although others concluded that public health practitioners must accept considerable responsibility for the deficiencies in public health. There was even dispute as to whether public health was, in fact, in disarray, given the substantial progress made in improving health status in the United States[63]. The Institute of Medicine's Report reinforces the central role of states but without adequately addressing the need for federal leadership and planning (Box 8.1)[63]. The bulk of funding for public health comes from federal sources; most public health problems are national in scope and do not respect administrative boundaries. The report did not prioritise recommendations and no evidence was produced to suggest that a structural reorganisation would improve function or outcome.

Practical recommendations to strengthen the public health system in five key areas include improvements in:

- the professional knowledge, skills and abilities of the public health workforce;
- the ability of individual public health officials and their agencies to provide dynamic community leadership;
- the ability of public health workers to access relevant information;
- the ability of public health organisations to engage with the community in planning, priority setting, and constituency building; and
- the ability of public health agencies to obtain and utilise fiscal resources[56].

8.4.3 Summary

Almost the entire debate on health care reform in the early 1990s centred on the financing and organisation of medical care. Public health was once

Box 8.1 HIV/AIDS: a public health challenge

The United States' response to the HIV-AIDS epidemic highlights the problems facing public health[63]. Although the HIV problem is huge, the public health response has not been in keeping with that given to other highly virulent, but less devastating, organisms. There was an absence of national leadership, and inadequate attention was devoted to the epidemic in its early stages; the main driving force of health policy was cost containment[64]. The extreme conservatism of mainstream United States politics in the 1980s limited the ability of the Centers for Disease Control to respond in a timely and appropriate fashion to the emerging epidemic leading to the charge that the Centers' programmes were afflicted by 'political correctness', rather than being guided by scientific knowledge[65]. The HIV epidemic came at a time when the public health structures within the United States were themselves suffering a 'wasting disease'[66]. Specific legislation may be required to protect the Centers for Disease Control from political interference in the future.

again marginalised[67]. The major lesson from the United States of America is that public health is unlikely to receive the attention and resources it requires until the delivery of personal medical services is organised more equitably. As long as state public health departments struggle to provide the medical care needs of millions of poor Americans, it is unrealistic to expect these agencies to focus seriously on public health issues. Furthermore, while the Federal Government continues to devolve responsibility for public health to the states, there is unlikely to be a coherent national approach to public health, especially with the Republican party firmly in control of Congress. The Republican Party stresses the importance of individual responsibility for public health issues and has reduced budgetary support for most of the federal agencies that perform a wide variety of public health functions[68]. The general antigovernment mood may lead to further reductions in essential government support for public health[69]. Public health professionals have failed to overcome the fragmentation of public health initiatives and build public support. Although there are some promising signs such as initiatives undertaken by schools of public health and local health departments and the increasing responsibility of managed care programmes for public health action, the outlook for public health in the United States of America is bleak. It is particularly disappointing that a country as wealthy as the United States shows such little leadership in public health.

8.5 Public health in Japan

From a public health perspective, Japan is of great interest. There have been tremendous improvements in life expectancy in Japan over the last 50 years and Japan now leads the international life expectancy tables. The rapid growth in wealth and the narrowing of the differences in its distribution, together with the typical diet with its continuing relatively low fat intake and recent decreases in salt intake, have all contributed to this favourable situation[70]. Health care is not likely to be a major factor. The public health system, in particular mass screening, may also have contributed, but is unlikely to be a major explanation, given the lack of convincing evidence on the effectiveness of screening for most non-communicable diseases.

Despite its long history of isolation and its unique cultural development, Japanese public health has been strongly influenced by Europe. The formal beginning of modern public health in Japan was the 1874 decree named Isei ('medical order') which was based on developments in Europe, especially Germany, and the United States of America[71]. The Isei consisted of 76 sections and covered a wide range of legislative needs, from public health administration to medical education. Regulations for the prevention of infectious diseases were promulgated in the late 1870s, stimulated by the need to control cholera and smallpox epidemics. From these beginnings, the responsibility for the prevention of infectious diseases rested with the city, town or village. Similarly, in 1890 the responsibility for construction of water supply systems was also decentralised although the central government provided strong direction.

After the devastation of the Second World War, the new constitution of 1946 stated that 'the state shall try to promote and improve the condition of social welfare and security, and of public health'[70] and the subsequent policies for public health were influenced by this constitutional requirement. The Medical Profession Law of 1948 stipulated that 'the physician shall contribute to improve and promote public health by performing medical care and health guidance, thereby maintaining the healthy livelihood of the nation'[72]. Environmental conditions in Japan deteriorated as industrial growth speeded up in the 1950s, and outbreaks of environmental poisoning led eventually to a new Ministry for the Environment in 1971.

Structurally, the Ministry of Health and Welfare is responsible for health administration, the Ministry of Education for school health, the Ministry of Labour for industrial health, and the Environmental Agency for control of environmental hazards. The Public Health Council, with its expert subgroups, advises the Minister of Health and Welfare. A variety of voluntary agencies play an important role in the delivery of public health services in Japan. Local voluntary organisations have been actively involved in public health campaigns associated with primary health care. Most new public policies and strategies are formulated by central government and implementation is delegated to local government. Preventive services are partly provided by prefectures, and partly by municipal governments. The national government provides between one-third and one-half of the cost of these activities. Public health, as defined by the constitution, also includes medical care, which is largely supplied by hospitals and clinics in the private sector.

A national network of health centres serves as the focus of public health activities including public health campaigns, health education activities, and health checks. The budget for health centres comes from national and local sources and each centre covers about 100 000 people. The range of activities of the health centre is very wide, and includes health education, personal advice on the prevention of disease, as well as maternal and child health guidance. Clinical treatment in the form of medications or operations are not included.

The major response of the Japanese Government to the emergence of non-communicable disease epidemics and the ageing of the population has been legislated requirements for periodic health checks and services for the elderly and an emphasis on health education activities. Mass screening especially for cancer, the leading cause of death, has been the major form of preventive activity in Japan for many decades. Mass screening for gastric cancer, the leading cause of cancer, is one of the major programmes supported financially by the 1982 Act for Health of the Elderly; also supported is screening for cervical cancer, breast cancer (including women as young as 35 years), lung cancer, and colon cancer. This act integrated health promotion and medical care for people aged over 40 years and provided financial support for medical cost for people aged over 70 years and to people aged 65–69 with serious handicap.

Health promotion programmes are conducted by municipal governments. The financial support for these programmes comes equally from the national, prefectural and municipal governments. The national health promotion programme is now in the third eight year phase. In the first and second five year programmes, primary and secondary prevention for cardiovascular disease and cancer detection and control were emphasised. Participation rates of screening have increased gradually. In the third eight year programme which began in 1992, integration of health promotion, medical care and social welfare is emphasised.

The incidence and death rates for gastric cancer are declining and it is commonly thought that health checks and mass screening have played an important part in this decline, despite the lack of convincing evidence on the value of screening. In 1988 nearly a third of the target population received health checks. An inverse relationship has been reported between the uptake of health checks in adults aged 40 years and over and hospital use by those aged 70 years and over[73]. The survey was based on data from all 509 Japanese cities with a population between 30000 and 200000. However, this ecological relationship is far from sufficient to indicate that the periodic health checks have been effective. Death rates from lung cancer are rising rapidly and will not respond to secondary preventive efforts.

Three major challenges face public health in Japan; the ageing population, the rise in the epidemic of tobacco caused disease, and the westernisation of the diet. Each challenge will require intersectoral collaboration on a scale not yet seen in Japan. The most likely explanation for the striking increase in life expectancy in Japan over the last half century is the increase in wealth, which has been distributed reasonably equitably. The dramatic declines in stroke deaths have been due to specific efforts to prevent high blood pressure, by lowering salt consumption in the entire population, and treatment programmes for hypertensive individuals. While it is impossible to specify the exact contribution of specific public health services to the dramatic improvement in life expectancy, it is clear that these services are not well equipped to deal with the major challenges now facing public health in Japan. The Japanese, however, do have more capacity to address problems more purposefully and with appropriate action than is apparent in most other countries.

8.6 Public health in Sweden

Sweden is included in this chapter because it is one of the most affluent countries in the world and has a strong reputation as an egalitarian state which pays particular attention to the welfare of its citizens. The Swedish health system has been under pressure since the late 1980s due to the poor growth rate of the Swedish economy, demographic changes, and concern with waiting lists and inefficiencies within the system[74]. As a consequence, the health system has been undergoing major structural transformation; the focus for change has been on medical care services, but public health has also been reorganised. A feature of the Swedish approach to health reform, and in contrast to reform in the United Kingdom and New Zealand, is the slow evolutionary nature of the process which involves extensive consultation[74,75].

From a historical perspective, it is noteworthy that a programme for public health in Sweden was initiated more than a 100 years before urbanisation and industrialisation gained momentum in the late nineteenth century[76]. In the second half of the eighteenth century, a variety of strategies were devised to increase the population which was deemed too small and in 1748 a system of national registration, on a parochial basis, was established to monitor population growth and other vital statistics. Nationwide disease registers and the systematic use of national registration numbers ensure that Sweden continues to offer exceptional opportunities for epidemiological research[77].

From an international perspective, health status in Sweden is very high, with low infant and maternal mortality rates and a high life expectancy. Inequalities in health are present as in all other countries, although the gradients are not as great as, for example, in the United Kingdom[78]. During the 1980s, however, smoking differentials by social class increased[79], and social class gradients for all cardiovascular risk factors have recently diminished among men but increased among women[80].

The county councils were established in the 1860s, mainly to operate hospitals. Their health care tasks have expanded over time and in the mid-1960s they took over from central government the responsibility for outpatient and general practitioner services and psychiatric care. The Health and Medical Services Act of 1983 extended still further the areas of responsibility of the county councils. Health care now accounts for 75–80% of the total expenditure of most county councils. The Act requires county councils to plan the development and organisation of the health and medical care needs of the entire county population.

Three of the largest municipalities, each with a population ranging from about 0.5 to 1.5 million, and 23 county councils have responsibility for health care. Responsibility for social welfare services and environmental health rests primarily with the municipalities, which number 281 and have populations ranging from about 5000 to 700000. Private health care has until recently existed only on a limited basis, with about 5% of physicians working full time in private practice.

Health and medical costs have increased very rapidly in recent decades, climbing during the last 15 years by 15–20% annually in current prices. The proportion of the GNP spent on health care reached a peak of 9.1% in 1983–84 but had declined to 7.1% by 1994. Health and medical care is financed by proportional income taxes levied by the county councils; between 1960 and 1984 the average county tax increased from about 4.5% to 13% and these taxes now cover 60% of the health and medical care costs with the remainder coming from a variety of state subsidies and funds from the national government.

The national government is responsible for ensuring that the health care system develops efficiently and in keeping with its overall objectives, based on the goals and the constraints of social welfare policy and macroeconomic factors. Central government administration is at two levels: the Ministry of Health and Social Affairs and the relatively independent administrative agencies, chiefly the National Board of Health and Welfare. This Board is involved in planning, monitoring and evaluating health and medical care, supervising the delivery of care and the performance of health care staff, and carrying out health information programmes.

In 1988 the Government appointed an advisory health policy group, the Public Health Group, to develop preventive health measures from a broad public health perspective. The Group serves in an advisory capacity on these matters to the Government and to the Health and Medical Care Advisory Committee, which was established to co-ordinate matters of health and medical care between the Government and the Federation of County Councils. The Group's duties also include taking independent, executive action to expedite measures in the public sector for improving public health. The Group has members from a variety of sectors including education, health and welfare, housing, food administration, environment, local authority, as well as from the public health and medical care sectors.

In 1991 the Public Health Group published a National Strategy For Health which proposed a comprehensive strategy for public health with a particular emphasis on counteracting health inequalities through preventive and health promoting measures[81]. The Report endorses the concept of 'sustainable development for health', in the same way as there is now a consensus on the importance of sustainable economic development. Unfortunately, the implications of this concept are not described. The Report suggests that public health efforts should increasingly be based on measures and programmes at the local level, particularly those involving active citizen participation. The Public Health Group suggested that the combined government effort to promote health would be made more effective by introducing explicit goals related to public health and equality throughout the public sector. This would require both a review of pre-existing goals and the formulation of new goals and should be implemented in connection with the overhaul of the relevant legislation. An important step is the development of methods for assessing the health impact of decisions and integrating this assessment into government decision, making use, wherever possible, of budgetary directives. This is an important new role for public health professionals in Sweden.

The Public Health Group recommended the formation of a Public Health Fund to subsidise or jointly finance developmental activities within various programme areas. It was suggested that the fund could be financed by a special charge on products hazardous to health. The fund was established, but from general tax revenue. Following another recommendation of the Public Health Group, an Institute of Public Health was established in 1992 to develop, stimulate and support health promotion and disease prevention activities at the national level. The main aims of the Public Health Institute are to support local and regional public health efforts and co-ordinate national efforts, develop research, and disseminate information.

Sweden has not yet developed a formal national health strategy, although it has adopted the WHO goal of a reduction in alcohol consumption by 25%. There are still no national and regional priorities. The Public Health Institute is in the process of preparing a full evaluation of public health in Sweden. A 1995 Report by the Health Care and Medical Priorities Commission recommended that cost efficient population based preventive interventions of documented effectiveness be of second priority (behind acute health care, care for immediately life-threatening disorders, and the care of patients with severe suffering and palliative terminal care)[82]. The implications of these priority rankings for resource allocation could be profound and their implementation will, no doubt, be difficult. The Swedish approach to health care priorities is distinctive in that it is led by politicians and represents a consensus[83].

Public health in Sweden has undergone considerable recent reorganisation, although the major emphasis has been on personal medical care services, driven, as usual, by cost considerations. The major challenge for public health in Sweden is to integrate national public health policies with the local delivery of public health services, which remain the responsibility of local authorities. Many county councils now have public health strategies, at least in embryonic form. The future of public health in Sweden depends to a large extent on whether the decentralised responsibilities can influence the public's health[84]. The impact of the recently introduced purchaser–provider split on public health programmes is yet to be assessed.

The evidence from other Scandinavian countries, for example Finland, on the power of local public health activities, is a cause for optimism. For example in North Karelia, major gains in the prevention and control of car-diovascular diseases were made as a result of intensive and co-ordinated local programmes. There was a synergy with national programmes and policies, but the local initiatives paved the way[85]. Local initiatives depend on the political persuasion of local governments and even in a relatively small country like Sweden there is a great variation in the emphasis given to public health among the counties. A real possibility as a result of the decentralisation of responsibility for public health, whether it be to states in the United States of America or counties as in Sweden, is that variations among regions will increase. An ideal approach would combine strong and progressive national guidelines, appropriate legislation and intersectoral support, with local initiatives and responsibilities.

8.7 Public health in New Zealand

The British colonisation of New Zealand which began in 1840 had a major influence on the evolution of public health although this was tempered by the different social and political environment in New Zealand. New Zealand has not experienced the problems associated with heavy industri-alisaton. As elsewhere, public health in nineteenth century New Zealand was primarily concerned with quarantine and sanitary reform. There was a general reluctance, however, to acknowledge mounting health problems in the colony and even epidemic outbreaks did not produce a sustained commitment to public health[86]. The Department of Public Health was established in 1901 in response to a plague scare and for a short time pre-vention was emphasised. In 1909, this Department was amalgamated with the Department of Hospitals and increasingly the focus shifted to hospital services, rather than the health of the whole population.

The social security legislation introduced by New Zealand's first Labour government in 1938 marked the origins of a health care system that was funded primarily by tax revenue and initially provided services free of direct charges. The power of the medical profession prevented the establishment of a national health service. Hospitals and public health services were administered separately with strong central direction until 1989 when 14 area health boards were charged with integrating the public health services (disease prevention and health promotion) and hospital services on a regional basis. Each board had a contractual arrangement with the Minister of Health to provide a comprehensive and integrated range of curative and preventive services with the overall aim of improving the health of the local population. With the publication of the Government's

Health Charter and National Health Goals and Targets in 1989, the health service for the first time began to plan coherently with a national focus but with devolved responsibility; priority was given to the reduction in inequalities in health status, especially the higher mortality and morbidity rates experienced by Maori which have their origin in long-standing socioeconomic inequalities[87].

In 1990, and driven by concern with the perceived rising cost of health care, the newly elected Conservative Government initiated radical changes to the health services[88]. These changes were one outcome of a voluntary, but radical, structural adjustment programme which had been initiated in 1984 by the Labour Government despite its traditional social democratic philosophy[89]. The organisation and delivery of public health services in New Zealand went full circle in a four year period, beginning in 1991. The major aims of the reforms were to introduce 'the market' into health services and to separate the purchasers of services from the providers.

The main proposal for public health was the separation of its funding and management from that of medical services. The Public Health Commission was established with responsibility for monitoring the state of public health, advising the Minister of Health on matters relating to public health, and for purchasing, or arranging for the purchase, of public health services. The justifications for the changes were the need to develop public health activities and to counter the diversion of resources from public health to medical services. After two years of preparation, the Public Health Commission was formally established in legislation in 1993 as a government agency outside the Ministry of Health. Public health services were purchased by the Public Health Commission with the four Regional Health Authorities (which replaced the 14 area health boards) acting as purchasing agencies at the regional level. Public health services were provided by the public health units of Crown Health Enterprises (the revamped hospitals) and other national providers, mostly non-governmental agencies.

The Public Health Commission had an independent board of seven directors and a statutory obligation to consult with members of the public and professional groups. It embarked upon a process of consultation on a scale never previously attempted in New Zealand in the field of public health. The state of the public health in New Zealand was thoroughly assessed in two annual reports[90]; special reports focused on the health of Maori and Pacific Island people living in New Zealand[91]. Policy advice to the Minister was published in a series of documents. The Public Health Commission had its own budget, less than 3% of the total health budget, of which 93% was spent purchasing services and 7% on information and policy advice. By contrast, in 1980 public funding for public health services was 6.5% of the total health expenditure and 4.2% in 1986[92].

The most important, and in the end critical, feature of the new arrangement was that the Public Health Commission was at arm's length from the Government. This distance encouraged the development of public health advice from a position of semi-independence. The success of this semi-independence depended crucially on the support of the Minister of Health. In its short existence, the Public Health Commission reported to three consecutive Ministers of Health, and only the first was explicitly supportive of the Commission.

In December 1994, after less than two years of formal existence, the Minister of Health announced plans to disestablish the Public Health Commission. The tasks of the Commission were taken over by the Ministry of Health in July 1995. The main reasons given for the change were the problems of co-ordination between medical and public health services and between non-regulatory and regulatory public health functions. It appears, however, that an underlying reason for the demise of the Commission was its semi-independent status as a Crown agency at arm's length from the Ministry. Despite the emphasis on 'contestable' advice in the market orientated health sector, the Government appeared uncomfortable receiving such advice from the Public Health Commission. It is hard to escape the impression that a major reason the Commission was abolished was its tendency to provide the government with advice contrary to the interests of the powerful health damaging interests in New Zealand, for example the alcohol and tobacco industries[93].

The future of public health in New Zealand is uncertain. There is concern that the public health budget will again be used to support the increasing demand for medical services and that the skilled workforce built up by the Commission will be dispersed. The independent advice provided by the Board of the Commission will now become the responsibility of a National Advisory Committee which is concerned with the full range of health and disability services. The high profile public health leadership provided by the Public Health Commission will not be maintained by the Ministry of Health which is concerned, above all, with the high cost of medical services.

The reintegration of public health and medical services in New Zealand, in the context of the purchaser–provider split, presents special challenges to the public health community. If primary health care providers take the initiative at the local level, as is occurring in the United Kingdom, public health activities may become localised and fragmented. This trend will be facilitated by the large number of non-governmental agencies competing for public health service contracts; rational population based planning will become even more difficult.

Postgraduate public health education is now well established in New Zealand with Diploma and Masters programmes offered by two universities. In 1995, approximately 100 full time equivalent students were enrolled, mostly mature students from the public health service; less than one-quarter were medically qualified. Public health research has been a priority in New Zealand since the Health Research Council was formed in 1989 from the long established Medical Research Council; the Public Health Research Committee is on equal standing with a Biomedical Research Committee. The public health research work force is still relatively small, but training fellowships and small grant awards are available to encourage new researchers.

The New Zealand experiment, with a Public Health Commission separate from the Ministry of Health, must be viewed as a failure[94]. The ultimate evidence of this failure is the premature ending of the Public Health Commission because its semi-independent nature was seen as a threat to the Government. Public health in New Zealand has lost its independent agency, budget, and advocate, and is once again led by a small group within a Ministry which is concerned, above all, with medical care issues and cost containment. Independent public health policy advice to government is desirable, even if not always desired. The New Zealand experience suggests that the institutional base for such advice must be securely supported by all major political parties as well as by the public health community. Without strong support, the existence of semi-independent public health agencies will be precarious.

8.8 Conclusion

This review of the recent history and current status of public health practice in five wealthy countries indicates that none has solved the problem of how best to organise public health services.

The current state of public health organisation and services is subjectively summarised for these five countries in Table 8.1. There is little relationship between the public health capacities and policies and the health status indicators. In none of these countries has the public health profession played a central role in the recent health service reform debates. Where reorganisation of public health services has taken place, for example in the United Kingdom and New Zealand, the process has not been driven by a primary concern with population health levels and the outcome has not been a strengthening of the practice of public health.

Table 8.1 *The state of public health in five wealthy countries*

	United Kingdom	United States of America	Japan	Sweden	New Zealand
Public health status[95]					
Life expectancy, 1993 (years)	76	76	79	78	76
Infant mortality,1993 (/1000 live births)	8	8	5	6	9
Age/sex standardised death rates 1990–95 (/100 000)	516	520	420	452	526
Immunisation coverage DPT3, 1993 (%)	91	83	87	99	81
Socioeconomic indicators[96]					
Unemployment 1993 (%)	10.2	6.7	2.5	8.2	9.5
Ratio of income of highest 20% of households to lowest 20%, 1981–92	9.6	8.9	4.3	4.6	8.8
Public health capacities					
Science	++	++	+	++	++
Education	++	+++	+	++	+++
Research	++	++	+	+	+
Professional organisations	+	+++	+	+	+
Public health policies					
National plan	Yes	Yes	No	No	Yes
Finanical support	Low	Low	Low	Low	Low
Priority of prevention	Low	Low	Low	Low	Low

Key: +++ Strong, ++ Moderate, + Weak.

The major gains in health status in Japan over the last few decades have not been due primarily to public health programmes. Rather the driving force seems to have been economic growth and relative equality in income distribution; specific features of Japanese society have probably also contributed, for example the supportive social networks. In the United Kingdom, public health has been medically dominated and close to clinical medicine and health services delivery. In the United States of America, the public health service has been distracted by its major responsibility for the delivery of medical services to the poor, although public health in general in the United States of America is not medically dominated. In none of these countries has the public health profession emerged as a strong advocate for a broad definition of public health with a focus on the social and economic determinants of health and disease.

There are few positive lessons for poor countries from the current state of public health services in wealthy countries. Fortunately, there are important lessons to be learnt from several poor countries, as we see in the next chapter.

Chapter 8 Key Points

- The health status of populations within wealthy countries varies, as do socioeconomic indicators.
- There is no obvious relationship between the organisation and delivery of public health services and health status.
- In all five wealthy countries, public health services are of low priority compared with medical care services.
- In none of these countries have the public health professions emerged as key players in the health reform process.
- There are few positive lessons for poor countries from the current state of public health services in wealthy countries.

References

1. Powles JW, Gifford S. Health of nations: lessons from Victoria, Australia. *Br Med J* 1993; **306**:125–7.
2. Roemer MI. *National Health Systems of the World*, vol 1. New York: Oxford University Press, 1991.
3. Mosbech J. Provision of public health services in Europe. In: Holland WW, Detels R, Knox G (eds). *Oxford Textbook of Public Health: Influences of Public Health*. Oxford: Oxford University Press, 1991.
4. Powles, JW. Personal communication, 22 May 1995.
5. Rose G. *The Strategy of Preventive Medicine*. Oxford: Oxford University Press, 1992.
6. Hamlin C. State medicine in Great Britain. In: Porter D (ed.). *The History of Public Health and the Modern State*. Amsterdam: Editions Rodopi BV, 1994.
7. Gore SM. Bovine Creutzfeldt–Jakob disease? Failures of epidemiology must be remedied. *Br Med J* 1996; **312**:791–3.
8. Lewis J. *What Price Community Medicine? The Philosophy, Practice and Politics of Public Health Since 1919*. Sussex: Wheatsheaf Books, 1986.
9. Madeley R. Public health and paradigms. *J Pub Hlth Med* 1993; **15**:223–5.
10. *Report of the Royal Commission on Medical Education 1965–68*. London: HMSO Cmd, 3569, 1968.
11. Anon. Public health advocacy: unpalatable truths. *Lancet* 1995; **345**:597–9.
12. Committee of Inquiry into the Future Development of the Public Health Function. *Public Health in England*. London: HMSO, Cmd, 289, 1988.
13. Holland WW, Fitzsimons B, O'Brien M. 'Back to the future' – public health research into the next century. *J Pub Hlth Med* 1994; **16**:4–10.
14. Whitty P, Jones I. Public health heresy: a challenge to the purchasing orthodoxy. *Br Med J* 1992; **304**:1039–41.

15. Griffiths R, McGregor A. Public health services in the UK. In: Holland WW, Detels R, Knox G (eds). *Oxford Textbook of Public Health: Influences of Public Health*. Oxford: Oxford University Press, 1991.
16. Milner P. Unsettling times for public health. *J Pub Hlth Med* 1994; **16**:1–3.
17. Bhopal RS. Public health medicine and purchasing health care. *Br Med J* 1993; **306**:381–2.
18. Smith R. *Health of a Nation: The BMJ View*. London: *British Medical Journal* 1991.
19. McKee M, Lang T. Secret government: the Scott report. *Br Med J* 1996; **312**:455–6.
20. Beecham L. Public health doctors have a vital role, says report. *Br Med J* 1993; **307**:1515.
21. Jacobson B. Purchasers, professionals, and public health: criticisms of Abrams report are misdirected. *Br Med J* 1994; **308**:981.
22. Iliffe S. The retreat from equity: implications of the shift towards a primary care-led NHS. *Crit Public Hlth* 1995; **6**:36–42.
23. Bhopal R. Public health medicine and primary health care: convergent, divergent, or parallel paths? *J Epidemiol Comm Hlth* 1995; **49**:113–16.
24. Sheard S. Gagging public health doctors. *Br Med J* 1994; **309**:1643–4.
25. Benzeval M, Judge K, Whitehead M (eds). *Tackling Inequalities in Health: An Agenda for Action*. London: King's Fund, 1995.
26. Scally G. Public health medicine in a new era. *Soc Sci Med* 1996; **42**:777–80.
27. Klein R. Labour's draft election manifesto: a triumph of style over matter? *Br Med J* 1996; **313**:68–9.
28. Beecham L. A Labour government will raise public health profile. *Br Med J* 1996; **312**:711.
29. World Health Organization Regional Office for Europe. *Targets for Health For All*. Copenhagen: World Health Organization, 1985.
30. World Health Organization. *The Health of Europe*. Copenhagen: WHO Regional Publications European Series No. 49, 1993.
31. Farmer RG, Goodman RA, Baldwin RJ. Health care and public health in the former Soviet Union, 1992. *Ann Intern Med* 1993; **119**:324–8.
32. Field MG. The health crisis in the former Soviet Union: report from the 'post-war' zone. *Soc Sci Med* 1995; **41**:1469–78.
33. Chenet L, McKee M, Fulop N, Bojan F, Brand H, Hort A, Kalbarczyk P. Changing life expectancy in central Europe: is there a single reason? *J Pub Hlth Med* 1996; **18**:329–36.
34. Boys RJ, Forster DP, Jozan P. Mortality from causes amenable and non-amenable to medical care: the experience of eastern Europe. *Br Med J* 1991; **303**:879–83.
35. Jamrozik K. A glimpse at public health in Eastern Europe. *Aust J Publ Hlth* 1994; **19**:102–3.
36. Rissel C. Impressions of public health in Germany and Europe. *Aust J Publ Hlth* 1994; **19**:103–4.
37. Gellert GA, Kaznady SI. Melting the Iron Curtain: opportunities for public health collaboration through international joint ventures. *Br Med J* 1991; **302**:633–5.
38. Colomber C, Lindstrom B, O'Dwyer A. European training in public health. *Eur J Pub Hlth* 1995; **5**:113–15.
39. McKee M, Bojan F, Normand C. A new programme for public health training in Hungary. *Eur J Pub Hlth* 1993; **3**:60–5.

40. McKee M, White M, Bojan F, Østbye T. Development of public health training in Hungary – an exercise in international co-operation. *J Pub Hlth Med* 1995; **17**:438–44.

41. Weindling P. Public Health in Germany. In: Porter D (ed.). *The History of Public Health and the Modern State*. Amsterdam: Editions Rodopi BV, 1994.

42. Kolip P, Schott T. The Postgraduate Public Health Training Programs in Germany. In: Laaser U, de Leeuw E, Stock C (eds). *Scientific Foundations for a Public Health Policy in Europe*. Weinheim: Juventa, 1995.

43. Ramsey M. Public Health in France. In: Porter D (ed.). *The History of Public Health and the Modern State*. Amsterdam: Editions Rodopi BV, 1994.

44. Ashton J. Setting the agenda for health in Europe. *Br Med J* 1992; **304**:1643–4.

45. Allen P. The Treaty of Maastricht and public health. *Health Trends* 1992; **24**:5–6.

46. Joffe M. Recent initiatives by the European Union. A new opportunity for promoting health. *Br Med J* 1994; **308**:610–11.

47. Commission of the European Communities. *Commission Communication on the Framework for Action in the Field of Public Health*. Brussels: Commission of the European Communities (LO3L93/559), 1993.

48. Rogers A. Obstacle to EU public health initiative. *Lancet* 1995; **345**:507.

49. Joossens L, Raw M. Are tobacco subsidies a misuse of public funds? *Br Med J* 1996; **312**:832–5.

50. Robbins A. A Prague winter for public health. *Am J Pub Hlth* 1995; **110**:295–7.

51. Fee E. Public Health and the State: The United States. In: Porter D (cd.). *The History of Public Health and the Modern State*. Amsterdam: Editions Rodopi BV, 1994.

52. Fee E. The origins and development of public health in the United States. In: Holland WW, Detels R, Knox G (eds). *Oxford Textbook of Public Health: Influences of Public Health*. Oxford: Oxford University Press, 1991.

53. Omenn GS, Nathan RP. What's behind those block grants in health? *New Engl J Med* 1982; **17**:1057–60.

54. Reichman LB. How to ensure the continual resurgence of tuberculosis. *Lancet* 1996; **347**:175.

55. Hinman AR, Bradford WR. Public Health Services in the United States. In: Holland WW, Detels R, Knox G (eds). *Oxford Textbook of Public Health: Influences of Public Health*. Oxford: Oxford University Press, 1991.

56. Roper WL, Baker EL, Dyal WW, Nicola RM. Strenghtening the Public Health System. *Pub Hlth Reports* 1992; **107**:609–15.

57. Lalonde M. *A New Perspective on the Health of Canadians*. Ottawa: National Health and Welfare, 1974.

58. McGinnis JM. Setting objectives for public health in the 1990s: experience and prospects. *Ann Rev Pub Hlth* 1990; **11**:231–49.

59. Committee for the Study of the Future of Public Health. *The Future of Public Health*. Washington: National Academy Press, 1988.

60. Trevinor FM, Jacobs JP. Public health and health care reform: the American Public Health Association's perspective. *J Pub Hlth Pol* 1994; **15**:397–406.

61. Miller CA, Brookes Ef, DeFriese GH, Gilbert B, Jain SC, Kavaler F. A survey of local public health departments and their directors. *Am J Pub Hlth* 1977; **67**:931–9.

62. Brumback CL. The IOM Report, the future of public health. *J Pub Hlth Pol* 1990; **11**:106–9.
63. Annas GJ. Back to the future: the IOM Report reconsidered. *Am J Pub Hlth* 1991; **81**:835–7.
64. Fox DM. AIDS and the American health policy: the history and prospects of a crisis of authority. *Milbank Mem Fund Q* 1986; **64**:7–33.
65. Francis DP. Toward a comprehensive HIV prevention program for the CDC and the nation. *JAMA* 1992; **268**:1444–7.
66. Kuller LH, Kingsley LA. The epidemic of AIDS: a failure of public health policy. *Milbank Mem Fund Q* 1986; **64**:56–78.
67. Navarro V. The future of public health in health care reform. *Am J Pub Hlth* 1994; **84**:729–30.
68. Iglehart JK. Health policy report: politics and public health. *New Engl J Med* 1996; **334**:203–7.
69. Foege W. Preventive medicine and public health. *JAMA* 1995; **273**:1712–13.
70. Marmot MG, Davey-Smith G. Why are the Japanese living longer? *Br Med J* 1989; **299**:1547–51.
71. Tatara K. The origins and development of public health in Japan. In: Holland WW, Detels R, Knox G (eds). *Oxford Textbook of Public Health. Influences of Public Health*. Oxford: Oxford University Press, 1991.
72. Koizumi A. Development of public health in Japan. *Asian Med J* 1982; **25**:14–20.
73. Tatara K, Shinsho F, Suzuki M, Takatorige T, Nakanisch N, Kuroda K. Relation between use of health checkups by middle aged adults and demand for inpatient care by elderly adults in Japan. *Br Med J* 1991; **302**:615–18.
74. Ham C. Reforming the Swedish health services. *Br Med J* 1994; **308**:219–20.
75. Glennerster H, Matsaganis M. The English and Swedish health care reforms. *Int J Hlth Serv* 1994; **24**:231–51.
76. Johannisson K. The people's health: public health policies in Sweden. In: Porter D (ed.). *The History of Public Health and the Modern State*. Amsterdam: Editions Rodopi BV, 1994.
77. Adami H-O. A paradise for epidemiologists? *Lancet* 1996; **347**:588–9.
78. Leon D, Vågerö D, Otterblad Olausson P. Social class differences in infant mortality in Sweden. A comparison with England and Wales. *Br Med J* 1992; **305**: 687–91.
79. Rosen M, Hanning M, Wall S. Changing smoking habits in Sweden: towards better health but not for all. *Int J Epidemiol* 1990; **19**:316–22.
80. Branström I. *A cardiovascular community intervention project in Northern Sweden*, PhD thesis. University of Umeå, Sweden, 1994.
81. The Public Health Group. *A National Strategy for Health: Summary Report Series No 13*. Stockholm: Public Health Group, 1991.
82. The Ministry of Health and Social Affairs. *Priorities in Health Care. Ethics, Economy, Implementation*. Stockholm, Swedish Parliamentary Priorities Commission, 1995.
83. McKee M, Figueras J. Setting priorities: can Britain learn from Sweden? *Br Med J* 1996; **312**:691–4.
84. Ovretveit J. Purchasing for health gain: the problems and prospects for purchasing for health gain in the 'managed markets' of the NHS and other European health systems. *Eur J Pub Hlth* 1993; **3**:77–84.
85. Puska P, Tuomilehto J, Nissinen A, Vartiainen E. *The North Karelia Project.*

20 Year Results and Experiences. Helsinki, National Public Health Institute (KTL), 1995.

86. Bryder L. A New World? Two hundred years of public health in Australia and New Zealand. In: Porter D (ed.). *The History of Public Health and the Modern State.* Amsterdam: Editions Rodopi BV, 1994.

87. Beaglehole R, Davis P. Setting national health goals and targets in the context of a fiscal crisis: the politics of social choice in New Zealand. *Int J Hlth Serv* 1992; **22**:417–28.

88. Salmond G, Mooney G, Laugesen M. Introduction to health care reform in New Zealand. *Health Policy* 1994; **24**:1–3.

89. Kelsey J. *The New Zealand Experiment: A World Model for Structural Adjustment?* Auckland: Auckland University Press, 1995.

90. Public Health Commission. *Our Health, Our Future: The State of Public Health in New Zealand.* Wellington: Public Health Commission, 1993 and 1994.

91. Public Health Commission. *The Health of Pacific Islands People in New Zealand.* Wellington: Public Health Commission, 1994.

92. Muthumal D, McKendry CG. *Health expenditure trends in New Zealand, 1980–92.* Wellington: Ministry of Health, 1993.

93. Barnett P, Malcolm L. To integrate or de-integrate? Fitting public health into New Zealand's reforming health system. *Eur J Pub Hlth* 1998; **8**:79–86.

94. Armstrong W, Bandaranayake D. *Public Health in New Zealand: Recent Changes and Future Prospects.* Monograph No 1. Department of Public Health, Wellington School of Medicine, 1995.

95. World Health Organization. *The World Health Report 1995. Bridging the Gaps.* Geneva: World Health Organization, 1995.

96. United Nations Development Programme. *Human Development Report.* New York: Oxford University Press, 1995.

9

Public health organisation and practice in poor countries

9.1 Introduction

Poor countries demonstrate tremendous diversity from a public health perspective. Some, such as China and Cuba, have shown remarkable improvements in health status over a few decades. Others, especially in sub-Saharan Africa, lag far behind the rest of the world. Many of the poorer countries have suffered recent economic setbacks which have had negative impacts on health. In this chapter, the organisation and delivery of public health activities are described and analysed in China, Cuba and the state of Kerala in India. These countries are success stories in that they have each made major health gains and offer hope for other countries striving to find health at low cost[1,2]. This chapter ends with a discussion of the role of international agencies in promoting public health in Africa, the region most in need of effective public health programmes.

9.2 China: public health a political priority

The evolution of public health in China has, from a global perspective, more importance than developments in any other country. With an estimated population in 1995 of 1.2 billion, China accounts for over 20% of the world's population and almost one-third of the population living in poor countries.

The history of public health in China over the last half century is a cause for cautious optimism. Since 1949, when the People's Republic of China was established, social and economic changes have led to dramatic improvements in the health status of the Chinese people. Life expectancy more than doubled from 32 years in 1950 to 70.5 years in 1992[3]. China's success in improving the health of its people far exceeds what could be expected at its stage of economic development raising interesting questions about the relationships between development and health. Much of China's success has been attributed to the national health system and to improvements in the provision of safe water and sanitation, nutrition, education (especially of women), and family planning services[2].

Chinese medicine is probably the world's oldest body of continuous medical knowledge with a history of over 4000 years of observation and theory[4]. Many Chinese discoveries predated Western discoveries. For example, by the beginning of the sixteenth century, the Chinese had discovered the value of variolation for the prevention of the more serious, naturally acquired, form of smallpox. From China the technique was brought to Turkey and then to England at the beginning of the eighteenth century.

The outbreak of pneumonic plague in Manchuria in 1911 advanced the cause of western medicine in China; the Peking Union Medical College was established in 1916 with support from the Rockefeller Foundation. At this time, there were no national or municipal health services in China. A programme in public health was developed at the Peking Union Medical College, which between 1924 and 1942 trained (in English) only 313 graduates. The most impressive aspect of this public health work was a rural health programme in Tingxian. This scheme, although having little impact on the health of the villages because of the widespread poverty, was ahead of its time in training village health workers.

The health challenges facing the new People's Republic of China in 1949 were staggering. Preventive medicine, despite its honourable tradition, was non-existent in most of China, and modern therapeutic medicine was unavailable in rural areas where 85% of China's population lived. Four basic guidelines for the organisation of health care were specified at the first National Health Congress in 1950:

- medicine should serve the workers, peasants and soldiers;
- preventive medicine should take precedence over therapeutic medicine;
- Chinese traditional medicine should be integrated with western medicine; and
- health work should be combined with mass movements.

The last principle was put into action with dramatic effect[5]. One of the best known of many campaigns was aimed at eliminating the 'four pests', originally defined, although not in all areas, as flies, mosquitoes, rats and grain-eating sparrows. When the elimination of sparrows appeared to be ecologically unsound, other pests were substituted[4]. Campaigns against specific diseases were also mounted, for example schistosomiasis.

The basic concept of the mass health campaigns was the involvement of people in dealing with important health problems, a foreshadowing of the Ottawa Charter concept of empowerment, albeit within the constraints of Chinese society. The first campaign was launched in 1951 and over the next 30 years there were an average of four or five campaigns a year. These campaigns were conducted under the leadership of the 'National Patriotic Health Campaigns Committee' and required an effective political, administrative and economic network, and unpaid volunteer labour. Although the mass campaigns were dramatic, the rapid expansion of health services infrastructure also contributed to the control of epidemic and endemic infections[6]. The key organisations were the anti-epidemic stations which became the best staffed and organised component of the public health service. These units had responsibility for all aspects of disease monitoring and control.

China made considerable progress in the 1950s and 1960s in solving the problems of infectious disease epidemics and in the provision of safe water and sanitation. Progress was not linear. A major famine in 1958–61, due to policies that de-emphasised the rural sector and encouraged urban growth, and adverse climatic factors which resulted in a dramatic decline in grain output, was responsible for up to 30 million premature deaths[7]. This was the largest famine in human history and went almost unrecognised outside China; major international relief aid was not attempted or even requested. A similar, but less destructive, period of disruption took place during the Cultural Revolution of the late 1960s.

In the first decades of the People's Republic of China, there was an ongoing tension between the Communist Party leadership and the professionals within the Ministry of Public Health. This tension resulted in a fragmentation of responsibility for health care, which was most apparent during the Great Leap Forward (1957–58). Health services, however, remained almost entirely in the public sector and curative and preventive care were closely integrated. Of overriding importance in the rapid improvements in health status in China was the attention given to increasing literacy and the provision of adequate housing and nutrition, all based, at least in principle, on the notion of collective responsibility.

China has now experienced three decades of communist leadership inspired by Mao Zedong, and almost two decades of economic and structural reform since his death in 1978. The latest period of reform has improved living standards for many Chinese, although death rates differ markedly between urban and rural areas, with a substantial burden of sickness and premature death being especially apparent in poor rural areas[8].

The recent reforms, however, have dismantled much of the health and medical system inspired by the early Chinese leadership, including the co-operative medical system in rural areas and the 'barefoot doctor' system[9-11]. In most rural areas, health care has shifted to a fee-for-service system, although urban residents are generally covered by a state insurance system because of work related benefits[12]. After the modernisation reforms of the 1980s the emphasis in health care shifted to curative activities because, it is said, this is what families were willing to pay for under the new financial arrangements[6]. Preventive services suffered as the 'barefoot doctors' were retrained as 'village doctors'; maternal and child services were especially at risk.

Ageing of the population represents a major challenge for China, with 6% of the population now over 65 years of age. The family planning policy of one child families will have major long-term ramifications for the future care and support of the elderly, especially in rural areas. China's experience shows that population growth can be rapidly controlled, although this did require coercive measures in the 1970s and early 1980s. In 1979 the one child per family policy was introduced because the birth rate was again increasing. Public compliance with the policy has been strong, but the stated goal of stabilising the population at about 1.3 billion by the year 2000 seems unattainable. Another major health challenge facing China is the emerging non-communicable disease epidemics, especially the tobacco induced epidemics. It has been projected that there will be two million smoking related deaths each year by the year 2025[13]. An important environmental issue is the heavy pollution of many Chinese cities, from both industrial and household sources.

Chinese health policy has been remarkably consistent in providing substantial resources for health (in 1990 about 3.5% of GDP was allocated to health)[3], and emphasising prevention, with about 5% of the total health budget (and 23% of government health expenditures) devoted to disease prevention and public health generally[11]. Furthermore, appropriate training and multi-sectoral and integrated policies have been emphasised. Much preventive medicine in China is organised vertically, with central responsibility for specific disease control programmes. Separate programmes are all administered by the epidemic prevention stations of the provincial and county health bureaus and this encourages integration. As non-communicable diseases become more important, increasing per capita income is likely to cease having beneficial effects on life expectancy. Control of the non-communicable disease epidemics will require changes in the training of health personnel and new public policies. Inevitably, the success of the preventive efforts has increased the demand for curative care. The preventive approach is not as prominent with non-communicable diseases as it was with communicable diseases, although smoking control programmes are belatedly being initiated.

It is too early to assess the impact of the recent and continuing reforms on public health in China. The approach adopted by the Chinese to the new public health problems, especially the non-communicable diseases, will be of great interest. The priority given to health in the early post-revolutionary era and the willingness to allocate resources to effective programmes, along with economic gains, had a huge impact on the health of Chinese. This occurred principally by reducing infectious diseases mortality and controlling population growth. It remains to be seen whether the modern Chinese health system will be able to cope so effectively with the current health challenges and whether health inequalities within China will increase.

9.3 Cuba: public health at all cost

Cuba is home to about ten million people and possesses some of the most favourable health indicators in the Americas. Cuba's overall achievements in health, education and general social and economic development since the overthrow of the old regime in 1959 have been remarkable. These successes are all the more impressive in the face of the enduring opposition of the United States of America which has, amongst other tactics, maintained a trade blockade. The Cuban experience indicates that population health status can be improved early on in the process of 'development'.

Some of Cuba's success can be attributed to the support of the former Soviet Union. More important, however, has been the priority given to health by the Cuban government. Public health according to President Castro 'became a challenge and a battleground between imperialism (United States of America) and ourselves, . . . and this multiplied our efforts. That is why we have developed this field and are striving to become a medical power with the best possible health indices'[14].

Cuba's achievements are now under severe threat. The tightening United States trade embargo, the collapse of the main trading partners in Central and Eastern Europe, and natural disasters, have created a situation of increasing scarcity. This situation threatens not only the health system, and the health of all Cubans, but also the government itself. Cuba is now in a period of uncertainty which will inevitably have adverse health effects. These threats highlight Cuba's public health achievements over the last three decades.

The trade embargo of the United States of America was first imposed in 1960 and since then has been implemented to varying degrees[15]. The United States 'Cuban Democracy Act of 1992' reimposed third-country sanctions that had been rescinded in 1975, thus prohibiting United States subsidiaries in other countries from trading with Cuba. Of the various factors causing difficulty for Cuba in the 1990s, the embargo is the only deliberate factor and is the only one that could, in the interests of the health of Cubans, be easily reversed. Unfortunately, the prospects for such a reversal are slim, at least in the short term.

The extent of Cuba's achievement in health are reflected in the health statistics which are now reliable[14]. In 1960, life expectancy at birth was 64 years and the infant mortality rate was 65 per 1000 live births. In 1993, life expectancy at birth had increased to 76 years and infant mortality was down to 14[16]. By comparison, life expectancy at birth in the United States of America was 76 years in 1993 and infant mortality was 9 per 1000 live births. So at least, in terms of life expectancy, Cuba has reached its goal of parity with the United States. It is doubtful, however, that this equality will be maintained in the face of the social and economic problems now facing Cuba.

The health advances have been achieved despite the poverty of Cuba. The GNP of Cuba per capita in 1992 in US dollars was estimated to be 1170, about one-twentieth that of the USA[17]. Even under the most difficult economic constraints, the Cuban government has made health a top priority, both because of its concern for Cubans and for symbolic reasons.

Despite Cuba's success in the health field it is unlikely that other poor countries will wish, or have the resources, to emulate Cuba's health systems. Cuba developed a health system in which primary health care was based on the central role of physicians. Furthermore, there has been a strong emphasis on expensive technology. This approach could only be developed under a political system in which decision making was highly centralised and planned and in which health commanded a high level of resources.

Primary health care in Cuba was initially based on polyclinic teams of physicians and nurses and other health workers which provided services for a defined population of between 25000 and 30000 people. The teams worked to guidelines established by the Ministry of Public Health and the collection and computerisation of statistical data on the population served was encouraged. The teams were to focus on prevention, but in practice there was too little time for preventive work[14]. In an effort to solve this and other problems with primary health care, the Cuban Government established the Family Doctor Programme as the central component of the medical system, beginning with a pilot project in 1984. This programme aimed to integrate primary health care with the community by putting a doctor and nurse team on every city block and in every rural community. A central task of the team is to monitor the health of the entire population, not just the sick, with each team responsible for between 120 and 150 families or about 600–700 people[14]; in most poor countries this ratio would be much greater. By 1991, the Family Doctor Programmes scheme covered over 60% of the population.

The major causes of death and disease in Cuba are now the non-communicable diseases, especially heart disease and cancer. A focus of the Family Doctor Programme is, therefore, on non-communicable disease risk factors, especially smoking, obesity, nutrition and physical inactivity. The top priority of the Family Doctor Programme has been the use of health education and popular participation in the implementation of health programmes. Health education takes place through lectures and the media, as well as at the individual level. To combat physical inactivity, the government promoted individual and group exercises and sports. One of the few benefits of the economic crisis of the 1990s is the increase in regular physical activity as a result of fuel shortages.

High levels of smoking present particular problems for the Cuban government because tobacco is an important export crop. Cuba is the second largest producer of tobacco in Latin America, after Brazil, and tobacco is second to sugar as a source of foreign exchange. In 1970, half the adult population (15 years and over) smoked regularly (two-thirds of men and one-third of women). In 1980, the pattern was unchanged despite non-smoking being encouraged since 1960. The most recent campaign began in 1986 and was assisted by a reduction in the availability of tobacco products in the early 1990s as part of the economic austerity programme. By 1990, 36% of the adult population was reported to be smoking regularly (49% of men and 25% of women)[18]. As in other countries, smoking is more prevalent among people with the least education, although the gradients are less than in many rich countries[19].

Mass participation in public health programmes in Cuba has been used to great effect. For example the campaign against haemorrhagic dengue fever in the early 1980s relied for its success on mass participation to eradicate the mosquito vector. Few other countries, apart from China, have demonstrated such an ability to mobilise the population to combat epidemic disease.

The public health approach to non-communicable disease prevention adopted by the Cuban Government raises interesting questions[20]. In particular, there are many similarities between the emphasis on health education of individuals in Cuba and most other countries. The anti-smoking campaign, for example, focuses on education and information, but not apparently on other important policy instruments such as taxation, although cigarettes have not been advertised in Cuba since 1960. Since 1971, tobacco has been marketed in two ways: on the rationed market, where the prices are kept low, and on the open market where prices are high. It is forbidden to sell cigarettes to people under the age of 16 years[19]. Recently legislative reforms have been introduced to restrict smoking in public places. The Cuban approach to disease prevention, involving health education and mass participation, is more equitable than in other countries because of the relatively equal distribution of goods and services in Cuba. Power in Cuba resides firmly with the Government, although much responsibility for health is devolved to the citizens.

The difficulties faced by the Cuban Government in providing adequate food and services for the people will lead to questioning of the Government's legitimacy. In some ways, it is a surprise that the Government has survived for so long after the collapse of its trading partners in Central and Eastern Europe. No doubt its long success in meeting the health needs of the people is part of the explanation for the Government's ability to maintain control. One manifestation of the difficulties facing Cuba is the epidemic of optic and peripheral neuropathy which began in 1991 and subsequently affected approximately 50 000 people, about 0.5% of the population[21]. The cause of the epidemic is probably a nutritional deficiency. Most patients are adults between the ages of 15 and 65 years, suggesting that children and old people are protected by their larger rations of milk and eggs. In typical Cuban fashion, a massive mobilisation of resources was undertaken to deal with the epidemic, including experts from the United States of America. Beginning in May 1993, the entire population received multi-vitamin tablets daily to overcome the possible nutritional deficiency and it appears that the epidemic has subsided[21].

Regrettably, it is unlikely that the unique health system built up over the last three and half decades will survive if the Government should fall. If the Cuban health and social system crumbles, the health of Cubans will deteriorate and health inequalities increase, as occurred in Central and Eastern Europe following the collapse of the Soviet Union.

9.4 Kerala State: public health at low cost

Kerala, a state in the south west of India, is discussed because of the contrast it provides to the rest of the Indian subcontinent. The health of

Keralites is considerably better than might be expected based on the enduring poverty of the state. The public health situation of Kerala is all the more remarkable when it is put into the context of India as a whole.

Modern public health in India is strongly influenced by the colonial experience. The system is geared to the priorities of the Government and is remote from the bulk of the population and inappropriate to many of their needs[22]. The provision of public health services in British India grew out of, and continued to be shaped by, anxieties aroused by the Indian mutiny of 1857. A strong driving force was the unhealthy state of the British troops[23,24]. The public health infrastructure evolved as one response to these concerns, but the emphasis was always on the needs of the military. Although the British were of the impression that they had done much to improve the health of Indians, there was a huge gap between the rhetoric and the reality[22]. This pattern was repeated by other colonising nations[25].

Despite British rule, India continued to be ravaged by major epidemics which led to negative population growth; between 1896 and 1914 bubonic plague killed over eight million people; malaria and tuberculosis killed more than twice as many over a similar period and the influenza epidemic of 1918–19 was even more devastating. The plague epidemic evoked fear and panic not caused by other epidemics[26], especially as control measures had little impact on the epidemic. By its inaction in the face of these epidemics, the colonial government missed the opportunity of adopting a broad public health approach based on sanitary measures, which was used successfully in many other countries[24]. By contrast, the plague outbreak of 1994 was more remarkable for the fear it generated, rather than the deaths caused[27,28], although the root cause was the same[29].

The reasons for the slow progress with public health in India were many[23]. British rule had itself created many health problems. For example, the military expeditions of the early nineteenth century contributed to the spread of cholera and agricultural developments disrupted traditional systems of drainage, exposing large tracts of the country to malaria. Furthermore, there was little consensus among colonial officials concerning medical policy in India. Medical experts contributed to the disagreements; the longstanding dispute over the control of malaria (mosquito eradication and general sanitation versus quinine prophylaxis) reinforced the limited desire for vigorous action[24,30].

Improvements in public health in British India depended on resources and co-operation between colonial officials and Indians. Neither the government nor key sections of the local population demonstrated the necessary long-term commitment to the provision of effective sanitary measures[26]. Public health in India under British rule must be judged a qualified failure, with only Europeans and a small sector of the Indian urban population receiving benefits. Unfortunately this legacy persists[22].

Kerala State was formed in 1956, in part from two 'native' states (Travancore and Cochin) which traditionally had considered the provision of health care facilities a primary duty of the Maharajah. The northern part of Kerala, previously part of Madras, lagged behind the rest of the state in health status. Infant mortality, for example in the north of Kerala was about twice as high as the rest of Kerala in 1956[31]. Of great interest is the extension to the whole of Kerala of the policies which had been successful in Travancore and Cochin and which produced similar outcomes within 35 years[31].

In 1991 Kerala's population was 29 million, under 4% of India's total population[31]. For many years Kerala has differed markedly from the rest of India in having an overall more favourable overall health profile[32]. Table 9.1 shows the comparative data for infant mortality rates, life expectancy at birth, and literacy rates for men and women[17,33]. Until the 1920s, infant mortality rates were similar to the rest of India[31,34]. Since then, the infant mortality rates have been consistently lower in Kerala and have declined much more rapidly. Similarly, life expectancy at birth has been higher and has increased more than in India as a whole since 1961.

Literacy rates, especially in women, are now much higher in Kerala than in India as a whole and the sex difference in literacy in Kerala is very small. A matriarchal caste in Kerala was historically particularly interested in the education of women and by the end of the nineteenth century every village in Kerala reportedly had a school. Other social and economic indicators do not, however, show Kerala to be at any advantage in comparison with other states. For example the per capita income for Kerala for the year 1981–82 ranked 11th among the Indian states and the percentage below the poverty line in 1977–78 was estimated to be 47 for Kerala and 48 for India as a whole; in 1987–88, 32% were estimated to be below the poverty line[31]. In 1991, the per capita domestic product was US$200 in Kerala and US$225 in India as a whole[17]. Modest increases in per capita income which occurred in Kerala through remittances from migrant workers in the Middle-Eastern Gulf countries, were complemented by social policies[31].

The nutritional intakes of Keralites also appear to be very similar to the rest of India[34]. Safe water supply coverage in Kerala is less than for the rest of India; in 1981, 37% of the villages in the State still lacked a safe water supply, more than twice the average of the other states. Per capita government expenditure on health care in Kerala, however, has been one of the

Table 9.1 *Literacy rates, infant mortality rates, and life expectancy at birth, Kerala and India, 1961–91*

	Kerala				India			
	1961	1971	1981	1991	1961	1971	1981	1991
Literacy rates (%)								
Men	65	77	85	94	34	40	–	53
Women	39	54	66	87	13	18	25	32
Infant mortality rates per 1000 live births	66	61	37	17[a]	114	138	119	83[a]
Life expectancy at birth								
Males	46.2	60.5	60.6	66.9	41.9	46.4	54.1	60.6
Females	50.0	61.1	62.1	72.8	40.6	44.7	54.7	61.7

[a] 1992

highest among all Indian states. The achievement of Kerala in human development would not have occurred without the commitment of financial resources by the State Government; as in China, international aid agencies played only a minor role.

The gains in infant mortality have been attributed to the expansion of immunisation programmes and possibly to an expansion of health facilities in the northern region[35]. The explanation for the overall better health experiences in Kerala is more complex. The role of health care has been strongly influenced by the level of education and health consciousness, especially of women; schooling encourages pupils to identify with the whole modern system, including health centres and the treatments they recommend[2].

The emphasis on rural, primary and female education has historically been greater in Kerala and this continued post-Independence. The high degree of literacy in Kerala is due to both government policy, which especially influenced the timing at which particular groups of people became literate in Kerala, and cultural attitudes towards women and women's attitudes about themselves which encouraged the acquisition of literacy[36]. Education is not merely a proxy for wealth. Education seems to have its impact on health by changing expectations and raising awareness, as much as by a direct impact on the behaviour of mothers[37]. With greater education and independence, mothers make more decisions more rapidly. Educated mothers are more likely to ensure a healthier distribution of food on a year round basis and utilise appropriate health[38]. Even so, a child of an uneducated mother living in a highly educated society has a much better chance of survival than a child of an educated woman living in a largely uneducated society[38], indicating the critical influence of social context on the absolute level of risk.

Unfortunately, it is not easy to reproduce in other countries the complex social, cultural and political circumstances that have generated a high degree of political awareness and the educational structure of Kerala. Education is no magic bullet; an effective and accessible health system is also required. Kerala provides several important lessons for other poor countries. Within a surprisingly short time, the quality of life for the broad majority of Keralites has improved, demonstrating that high levels of health and social development can be achieved in the absence of high rates of economic growth. Kerala's success occurred within the context of a country which has been notably unsuccessful in its attempts to achieve a similar improvement in quality of life for its citizens using conventional western approaches, such as medical care services and family planning programmes. Kerala's success is a result of a particular set of mutually supporting and reinforcing factors, not just education or 'political will', with equity considerations being of fundamental importance[2]. The Kerala experience indicates that vigorous public action can transform the level of social development and cause major improvements in social and health indicators, even at relatively low levels of per capita income and within a single generation.

9.5 Africa: poor health at high cost

Africa is a huge continent comprising over 50 nations with a total population of approximately 600 million, including 500 million in sub-Saharan Africa. The history of Africa's self-development, before foreign rule began, is impressive[39]. Africa now faces a remarkable range of complex problems whose origins are many and varied. Responsibility for much of the present crisis in Africa lies within the nation states, which in turn were a creation of the colonial powers and the 'tribes' they empowered, as Africa began to emerge from colonial rule in the 1950s[39].

The slave trade devastated Africa, especially West Africa, for almost two centuries. This trade was one of the precursors of deteriorating health standards and social breakdown in Africa, although it undoubtedly contributed to the rising standard of living in Europe[40]. Further destruction of African society took place after the colonial partition in the 1880s[41]. The continuing transfer of wealth to the rich countries of the north, environmental degradation, natural disasters, harsh governments and dictatorships, and civil strife, have compounded Africa's problems over the last half century. Disease epidemics, of which AIDS is the most recent, have added to the African misery.

From a public health perspective, all is not despair. Despite its social, economic and political problems, the health of most Africans has improved; however, in comparison with all other countries, African countries are towards the bottom of the health tables. For example in 1992 life expectancy in 20 African countries was still less than 50 years, although in almost all African countries life expectancy increased over the last three decades. Birth rates and infant mortality rates in Africa are amongst the highest in the world. Improvements have occurred in all countries, although periods of deterioration, especially since 1980, have resulted in infant mortality rates in some countries being only a little better in the early 1990s than the rates in the mid-1960s. For example, in Uganda in 1965 the infant mortality rate was 121 per 1000 live births; in 1993 it was still over 100[16]. Adult mortality rates in sub-Saharan Africa are difficult to ascertain in the absence of accurate mortality statistics. Where data are available, the situation is bleak. For example, in a rural district in Tanzania in the period 1992–95, mortality was over 40 times higher in 20–24 year old women than in the same age women in England and Wales[42].

During the 1960s and 1970s considerable progress was made in promoting education and health care; child mortality rates more than halved between 1960 and 1990, an achievement that took more than a century in Europe. The late 1970s and 1980s, however, was a time of severe economic crisis, precipitated by rises in oil prices, increasing interest rates, a reduction in prices for exports from poor countries, and a fall in tax revenues. Poor countries had to borrow on the international market to continue to govern; debt servicing requirements increased dramatically, and by the early 1980s many countries in Africa were unable to meet these repayments. Structural adjustment programmes were designed by the World Bank and the International Monetary Fund to overcome these difficulties in return for debt rescheduling[43,44].

Structural adjustment programmes are now in place in many poor countries, not just in Africa. Most debt relief and overseas aid are now dependent on recipient countries agreeing to these programmes[44]. The imposition of these programmes by agencies such as the World Bank and the International Monetary Fund is one indication of the recent ascendancy of these agencies over health affairs in Africa; the World Health Organization has been relegated to a subsidiary role[45].

Structural adjustment programmes include a wide range of measures:

trade liberalisation, currency devaluation, increased interest rates, introduction of user charges for medical care, and a decrease in spending on
social welfare programmes. The ultimate aim is to stimulate economic
growth. The evidence on the impact of these programmes on long-term economic growth is debatable, although a few countries, especially in South
America, have responded positively – at least in the short term.

There is, unfortunately, little doubt that structural adjustment has had
an adverse short-term effect on the health of many people in poor countries
as a consequence of rising prices, increasing unemployment and cuts to
health services. Child mortality rates have risen in the late 1980s in several
African countries, malnutrition has increased, and several endemic diseases
have become more prominent[45]. It is difficult to blame structural adjustment for all these problems but popular discontent, the so called 'IMF food
riots', has been directed at the international agencies; many non-governmental aid agencies have been strongly critical of structural adjustment[45].

The colonial powers extracted great wealth from their colonies. Money
has continued to move from poor countries in the South to rich countries
in the North. In 1992, for example, there was a net flow of US$19 billion
from the 40 poorest countries in the world to the richest. These poor countries, 30 of them in sub-Saharan Africa, received $16 billion in aid, but paid
$35 billion in debt repayments and interest. They defaulted on $12 billion
which was added to their debt which reached $450 billion[45].

While spending on health and other social services has been reduced,
military spending has increased and armies continue to flourish in Africa,
in the midst of human misery. Efforts to balance government budgets were
not unfortunately directed to reducing military spending; social services
were an easier target. It is estimated that in sub-Saharan Africa in 1991,
$8 billion was spent on arms with high military spending continuing among
very poor countries such as Sudan, Ethiopia, Chad, Burkina Faso,
Mozambique and Mali[46]. Much of the blame for this spending rests with
rich countries which have not done enough to phase out military assistance
or arms sales[47]. The United States of America and the former Soviet Union
accounted for over half of the export trade in military equipment; encour-
agingly, the total value of the trade in 1992, US$18 billion, was less than
half the 1988 figure[46].

The steps required to ease the immediate economic problems in Africa
are straightforward. Of most importance is the removal of the crushing
debt. By 1993 only 3% of total African debt had been cancelled[44]. The
World Bank and International Monetary Fund debt can not be cancelled
for constitutional reasons, only its repayment delayed. Unfortunately,

prospects for debt relief are not great. No concrete progress on this issue was made at the 1995 United Nations World Summit for Social Development which considered proposals for the reduction of global poverty, now encompassing more than one billion people[48]. Wealthy nations reiterated their belief that free trade and deregulation will lead to economic growth which in turn will reduce global poverty; poor counties resented being told what to do. One positive step was acceptance of the '20/20 initiative' which calls on donor and poor countries to increase their spending on basic social services, including health services, to 20% of total official development assistance, and 20% of national budgets, respectively. It remains to be seen whether this agreement will be implemented.

The second step is to ensure that economic restructuring puts the needs of poor people first, especially their needs for health and education. The World Bank is apparently changing its policy and giving more emphasis to health and social issues, although the impact of these changes has yet to be felt[44]. Public support for these measures is vital. Health professionals have a key role to play, given the impact of structural adjustment on health. Of equal importance to short-term economic reform is the need to rebuild African societies. In the long-term, the politics of mass participation offer the most hope for overcoming the ongoing strife that affects Africa[39]. The prospects for much of Africa remain bleak; however, there is cause for cautious optimism. In 1993 the apartheid regime in South Africa came to a surprisingly peaceful end, although the public health challenges remain formidable[49].

9.6 Conclusion

The experience of Kerala and China and a few other countries such as Sri Lanka and Costa Rica, which have achieved high levels of population health at relatively low cost, indicates that unusually low mortality can be achieved if several conditions are met[2]. Sufficient female autonomy is a prerequisite and this in turn is strongly influenced by the dominant culture. Many of the countries which have performed, from a health perspective, below that expected on the basis of their national wealth are Moslem, a religion which, in general, does not support female autonomy. Religion is not, however, an absolute barrier to progress because some eastern Moslem countries, such as Malaysia, have achieved a better health status than would be expected on the basis of per capita income. Adequate levels of nutrition are another prerequisite. Sufficient resources must also be devoted to the public health infrastructure and to efficient and accessible health services and education, especially for females. Preventive health services must be available, for example childhood immunisation and pre and post-natal services.

Political consensus on the priority of high levels of education and health is a central requirement. This does not require a broad consensus on all political issues, only that successive governments are not able to overturn the advances of their predecessors. The central role of policy analysis in reforming the health sector in poor countries requires more attention[50]. Above all, it is clear from the poor countries which have made rapid gains in health status that progress will not occur as a byproduct of economic growth. Government leadership at national and regional levels is essential and must take precedence over the operation of market forces[2]. Unfortunately, in most countries of the world today, this lesson has not yet been learnt.

Chapter 9 Key Points

- Most poor countries have poor health statistics.
- A few poor countries have achieved remarkably good health statistics at relatively low cost.
- The experience from these countries suggest the following conditions are required:
  - political consensus on the high priority of education and health services;
  - female autonomy;
  - readily available education, especially for women;
  - adequate nutrition; and
  - efficient and accessible health services, including preventive services.

References

1. Halstead SB, Walsh JA, Warren KS (eds). *Good Health at Low Cost*. New York: Rockefeller Foundation, 1985.
2. Caldwell JC. Routes to low mortality in poor countries. *Pop Dev Review* 1986; **12**:171–220.
3. World Development Report, 1993 : *Investing in Health, World Development Indicators*. New York: Oxford University Press, 1993.
4. Sidel R, Sidel VW. *The Health Of China: Current Conflicts In Medical And Human Services For One Billion People*. Boston: Beacon Press, 1982.
5. Xu W. Flourishing health work in China. *Soc Sci Med* 1995; **41**:1043–5.
6. Taylor CE, Parker RL, Dong-Lu Z. Public health policies and strategies in China. In: Holland WW, Detels R, Knox G (eds). *Oxford Textbook of Public Health*. Oxford: Oxford University Press, 1991.

7. Ashton B, Hill K, Piazza A, Zeita R. Famine in China, 1958–61. *Pop Dev Review* 1984; **10**:613–45.
8. Lawson JS, Lin V. Health status differentials in the People's Republic of China. *Am J Pub Hlth* 1994; **84**:737–41.
9. Shi L. Health care in China: a rural–urban comparison after the socioeconomic reforms. *Bull WHO* 1993; **71**:723–36.
10. Chen X, Hu T, Lin Z. The rise and decline of the cooperative medical system in rural China. *Int J Hlth Serv* 1993; **23**:731–42.
11. Hsiao WCL. The Chinese health care system: lessons for other nations. *Soc Sci Med* 1995; **41**:1047–55.
12. Zheng X, Hillier S. The reforms of the Chinese health care system: county level changes: the Jiangxi Study. *Soc Sci Med* 1995; **41**:1057–64.
13. World Health Organization. *Tobacco Alert*. Geneva: WHO, April 1995:3.
14. Feinsilver JM. *Healing the Masses: Cuban Health Politics At Home And Abroad*. Berkeley: University of California Press, 1993.
15. Kuntz D. The politics of suffering: the impact of the US embargo on the health of the Cuban people: report of a fact-finding trip to Cuba, 6–11 June 1993. *Int J Hlth Serv* 1994; **24**:161–79.
16. World Health Organization. *The World Health Report 1995. Bridging the Gaps*. Geneva: World Health Organization, 1995.
17. UNICEF. *The State of the World's Children*. New York: Oxford University Press, 1995.
18. Data provided by AD Lopez. Personal communication, Geneva: 17 March 1995.
19. A Report of the Pan American Health Organization. *Tobacco or Health: Status in the Americas*. Washington DC, Pan American Health Organization/Pan American Sanitary Bureau: Regional Office of the World Health Organisation, 1992.
20. Tesh S. Health education in Cuba: a preface. *Int J Hlth Serv* 1986; **16**:87–104.
21. Centers for Disease Control. Epidemic neuropathy – Cuba, 1991–1994. *JAMA* 1994; **271**:1154–5.
22. Arnold D. Crisis and contradiction in India's public health. In: Porter D (ed.). *The History of Public Health and the Modern State*. Amsterdam: Editions Rodopi BV, 1994.
23. Harrison H. *Public Health in British India: Anglo-Indian Preventive Medicine 1859–1914*. Cambridge: Cambridge University Press, 1994.
24. Ramasubban R. Imperial health in British India, 1857–1900. In: MacLeod R, Lewis M (eds). *Disease, Medicine and Empire*. London: Routledge, 1988.
25. MacLeod R. Introduction. In: MacLeod R, Lewis M (eds). *Disease, Medicine and Empire*. London: Routledge, 1988.
26. Chandavarkar R. Plague panic and epidemic politics in India, 1896–1914. In: Ranger T, Slack P (eds). *Epidemics and Ideas: Essays on the Historical Perception and Pestilence*. Cambridge: Cambridge University Press, 1992.
27. Madan TN. The plague in India, 1994. *Soc Sci Med* 1995; **40**:1167–8.
28. John TJ. Final thoughts on India's 1994 plague outbreaks. *Lancet* 1995; **346**:765.
29. Cook GC. Plague: past and future implications for India. *Pub Hlth* 1995; **109**:7–11.
30. Worboys M. Manson, Ross and colonial medical policy: tropical medicine in London and Liverpool, 1899–1914. In: MacLeod R, Lewis M (eds). *Disease, Medicine and Empire*. Routledge: London and New York, 1988.

31. Krishnan TN. *The Route to Social Development in Kerala. Social Intermediation and Public Action: a retrospective study, 1960–1993*. New York: UNICEF, 1996.
32. Jeffrey R. *The Politics of Health in India*. Berkeley: University of California Press, 1988.
33. Gulati L. Population ageing and women in Kerala State, India. *Asia-Pac Pop J* 1993; **8**:53–63.
34. Nag M. The impact of social and economic development on mortality: comparative study of Kerala and West Bengal. In: Halstead SB, Walsh JA, Warren KS (eds). *Good Health at Low Cost*. New York: Rockefeller Foundation, 1985.
35. Krishnan TN. Health statistics in Kerala State, India. In: Halstead SB, Walsh JA, Warren KS (eds). *Good Health at Low Cost*. New York: Rockefeller Foundation, 1985.
36. Jeffrey R. Governments and culture: how women made Kerala literate. *Pacific Affairs* 1987; **60**:447–72.
37. Caldwell JC, Caldwell P, Gajanayake I, Orubuloye IO, Pieris I, Reddy PH. Cultural, social and behavioural determinants of health and their mechanisms: a report on related research programs. In: Caldwell J, Findley S, Caldwell P, Santow G, Cosford W, Braid J, Broers-Freeman D. *What We Know About Health Transitions*, vol 2. Canberra: Australian National University, 1990.
38. Caldwell JC, Reddy PH, Caldwell P. The social component of mortality decline: an investigation in South India employing alternative methodologies. *Pop Stud* 1983; **37**:185–205.
39. Davidson B. *The Black Man's Burden: Africa and the Curse of the Nation-State*. London: James Currey Limited, 1992.
40. Turshen M. *The Political Ecology of Disease in Tanzania*. New Brunswick: Rutgers University Press, 1984.
41. Kanji N, Kanji N, Manji F. From development to sustained crisis: structural adjustment, equity and health. *Soc Sci Med* 1991; **33**:985–93.
42. Kitange HM, Machibya H, Black J, Mtasiwa DM, Masuki G, et al. Outlook for survivors of childhood in sub-Saharan Africa: adult mortality in Tanzania. *Br Med J* 1996; **312**:216–20.
43. Godlee F. Third world debt: what's the point of immunising children if we are then going to starve them? *Br Med J* 1993; **307**:1369–70.
44. Logie DE, Woodroffe J. Structural adjustment: the wrong prescription for Africa? *Br Med J* 1993; **307**:41–4.
45. Godlee F. The World Health Organization in Africa. *Br Med J* 1994; **309**:553–4.
46. United Nations Development Programme. *Human Development Report*. New York: Oxford University Press, 1994.
47. Sidel VW. The international arms trade and its impact on health. *Br Med J* 1995; **311**:1677–80.
48. Logie D, Haines A. Copenhagen's challenge: to balance budgets without unbalancing lives. *Br Med J* 1995; **310**:544–5.
49. Geiger HJ. Letter from South Africa. *Publ Hlth Rep* 1995; **110**:114–16.
50. Walt G, Gilson L. Reforming the health sector in developing countries: the central role of policy analysis. *Hlth Pol Planning* 1994; **9**:353–70.

10

Public health at the crossroads

10.1 Introduction

Public health is at the crossroads; and not for the first time. In 1926 Winslow described public health in the United States of America as standing 'at the crossroads' because of challenges posed by the emergence of the epidemics of non-communicable diseases[1]. Winslow recommended a narrow path of early detection of disease with 'education of the individual in the principles of healthy living' as the desirable goal of public health.

From a historical perspective, there are strong parallels between the state of public health today and the situation at the end of the nineteenth century. Mid-nineteenth century epidemiology and public health were successful in controlling the epidemics of infectious diseases. Unfortunately, towards the end of the century epidemiology and public health lost their way and became dominated by bacteriology and the identification of high risk populations.

A similar cycle is now recurring. Following the successes in controlling the major non-communicable disease epidemics in many countries in the second half of this century, epidemiology and public health are in danger of succumbing to a new paradigm. Molecular and genetic approaches to the control of disease are gaining ground and influencing the research agendas. In both historical periods, a fundamental failing of the public health profession has been the inability of public health specialists to articulate and act upon a broad vision of public health and confront the underlying causes of premature death and disability.

As we approach the end of the twentieth century the public health movement is under threat in both wealthy and poor countries. Fortunately this also represents an opportunity for reinvigoration. This chapter summarises the challenges facing public health practitioners and the steps that need to be taken to move towards centre stage.

211

Table 10.1 *Two directions for public health*

Characteristics	Broad	Narrow
Definition of health	Foundations for health	Absence of disease
Underlying theory	Socio-structural	'Lifestyle'
Motivating concerns	Inequalities in health; poverty; global environmental issues	Individual risks of disease
Major public health activities	Linkage of public health sciences with policy making	Cost-containment; disease prevention, especially in high risk groups
Place of epidemiology	Balanced by other methods; participatory research	Emphasis on technique and clinical and molecular epidemiology
Advantages	Potential long-term global benefit	Short-term benefits
Disadvantages	Risk of failure because of breadth of concerns	Failure to address fundamental threats to global health

10.2 Public health: definitions and scope

Public health has always been pulled in two different directions: towards a broad focus on the underlying social and economic causes of health and disease and towards a narrow medical focus. These two pathways are summarised in Table 10.1.

Public health movements in most countries are heading down the narrow disease focused route under the influence of the prevailing social and economic ideology. Only a serious and concerted effort will divert public health to a broader perspective. Public health professionals will need to ensure that the alternative routes and their implications are widely debated and discussed. A failure to take this initiative will inevitably lead to further movement down the narrow public health pathway.

To be most effective, public health practitioners require a firm sense of identity based on a broad and inclusive definition of public health. A modified version of Winslow's definition of public health is suitably broad and inclusive: 'one of the collective efforts organised by society to prevent premature death, illness, injury and disability, and to promote the population's health'. The importance of this definition is that it includes medical care and rehabilitation, health promotion, and the underlying social, economic and cultural determinants of health and disease. Unfortunately, this definition has not been acted upon because medical care is usually seen as the solution to health problems.

The integration of medical care under the public health umbrella would facilitate the process of setting broad health goals and targets and encourage resources to flow to prevention. At the same time, public health specialists would contribute to the organisational aspects of universally accessible medical care and to the development of evidence based medicine.

There is tremendous potential for merging the two disciplines, public health and medical care, because both sets of activities are often under the direction of the same government department. The national health goals and targets movements of the late 1980s had the overall objective of redirecting medical care resources towards the achievement of public health goals[2]. Such a policy redirection requires strong political leadership and is more likely to achieve the desired ends if it has been motivated by a real desire to support public health and to strive for equality of opportunity for health rather than the need to legitimise cost containment.

An important task for public health practitioners is balancing effort devoted to controlling individual risk factors and dealing with the underlying social and economic causes of health. It is relatively easy to research a 'new' risk factor or to implement a high risk disease control strategy. It is much harder to develop an innovative research programme exploring the impact of income inequality on health or to present evidence based policy advice on income distribution. The latter requires input from many different social policy and public health scientists.

A refocusing 'upstream' involves a move away from a predominant concern with individual risks towards the social structures and processes which generate health and disease[3]. This is not to deny that there is still much to be gained from dealing with specific causes of premature death and disease using effective public health measures. For example, in many countries cigarette smoking is the most readily preventable cause of disease. The public health significance of smoking, however, is closely related to global and national economic, social and political issues. The complex reasons for the high rates of smoking by oppressed groups, including women, highlight the strong links between social forces and high risk behaviour[4].

Strategies that concentrate solely on the prevention of disease, for example screening, have associated costs which may divert resources from more fundamental health promotion activities. A resolution of the dilemma posed by the disease prevention – health promotion balance is yet to be achieved. Public health professionals, by explicitly recognising their chosen path of action, can assist in reaching the necessary balance.

Apart from a firm sense of direction, public health also requires a strong and clearly articulated theoretical foundation based on a clear appreciation of the history of public health, in order to avoid being at the mercy of the prevailing ideology. Progress in public health will be easier when there is a more sympathetic attitude towards collective endeavour.

Unfortunately, the term 'public health' is a source of confusion[5]. 'Public' can refer either to the action of individual members of the community or to the social groups of which individuals are part. The meaning adopted is critical for the practice of public health; different interpretations lead to the dominance of either individual or collective strategies. Regrettably, the individualistic interpretation and practice are currently dominant although public health is still underpinned in most countries by collective strategies such as garbage collection and clean water supplies.

Similarly, the meaning of 'health' is of central importance to the orientation of public health activities. If 'health' is equated with the absence of disease, as it is in much of epidemiology, then disease prevention will receive more emphasis. If, on the other hand, 'health' is interpreted in a broad sense, involving the equitable distribution of the foundations for health, health promotion will be emphasised[6]. A definition of public health based on a strong commitment to collective endeavour and a broad view of health will lead to public health activities quite distinct from a definition which emphasises the individualistic approach to health.

10.3 Recent public health movements

10.3.1 New public health

The term 'new public health', first used in 1916, is unfortunate because every generation can appropriate the term 'new'. Its original use referred to a narrow view of public health based on bacteriology[7]. Identification and treatment of individual carriers of tuberculosis was seen as the solution to this epidemic, rather than an improvement of living conditions of the whole population.

The most recent use of the term 'new public health' emerged from a recognition that major health problems cannot be solved by medical care[8]. This was most clearly articulated by the Lalonde Report from the Canadian Government, published in 1974 under the name of the then Minister of National Health and Welfare[9], which led the first wave of modern health promotion. The report proposed the 'health field concept' which included four elements: human biology, environment, lifestyle and health care organisation. This 'new perspective' aimed to direct more resources into a positive approach to health with greater emphasis on health promotion. Unfortunately, for a variety of reasons, not least the economic crisis of the late 1970s, most health promotion energy was diverted towards the 'lifestyle' health field, with health education as the favoured strategy.

The United States Surgeon General followed in 1979 with a report which led to an ambitious set of quantified health goals and targets for the year 1990[10]; most of the goals focused on disease prevention and emphasised individual lifestyle strategies[11]. Many other countries adopted a similar approach to health goals and targets, with health education being the prime strategy and cost containment the underlying motivation.

At a global level, the response of WHO was Health For All by the Year 2000, a proposal which recognised that the main determinants of health are outside the health care sector; primary health care was seen as the key to achieving this goal at the Alma Ata conference in 1978[12]. Primary health care, as originally formulated, stressed the importance of equity in access to community based services, and encouraged a comprehensive approach to improving health that included actions outside the health sector. It did not take long, however, for this comprehensive approach to be replaced by selective and targeted strategies to disease control such as childhood immunisation. Such vertical programmes rely heavily on specific and focused activities[13] and represent a major departure from the original Health For All concept[14].

10.3.2 *The Ottawa Charter: new dimensions to health promotion*

The Lalonde Report and related documents were criticised because of the perceived emphasis on victim blaming and the neglect of the social and economic determinants of health. In contrast, the Health for All proposal was rejected as being too ambitious. Out of these criticisms came the second wave of modern health promotion under the banner of the Ottawa Charter for Health Promotion, largely developed by the World Health Organization (Box 10.1)[15].

In comparison with the expansive Health for All proposals, the Ottawa Charter was strongly influenced by the more difficult economic environment of the 1980s. The Healthy Cities project, launched in 1986 as both a vision and a movement, has been one of the major instruments for the implementation of the Ottawa Charter[16]. Healthy Cities grew as a series of local community experiments, usually led by health promotion practitioners. Although some of these projects have achieved success and have been

---

Box 10.1   The Ottawa Charter and health promotion

The Ottawa Charter breaks health promotion into five action areas:

• building healthy public policy;
• creating supportive environments;
• strengthening community action;
• developing personal skills; and
• re-orienting health services.

The Ottawa Charter is primarily a philosophical document and it has not been easy to translate into practical use. The Ottawa Charter approach to health promotion down-plays the lifestyle (health education) approach to health and emphasises the importance of social structures and policy as key health determinants. Health is placed firmly in the sociopolitical domain, well outside the individual and biological realm. This major shift in focus has not been easy to apply in practice and the conceptual vagueness leads to difficulties in evaluation.

---

sustained, many more have struggled and by focusing on individual cities the wider social and economic and political factors have often been ignored[16]. In the final analysis, unless they are translated into policies, projects are only of limited value in demonstrating possible approaches to health promotion.

A reassessment of the Ottawa Charter is overdue because of the difficulty of implementing its five components and the perceived authoritarian nature of much of modern health promotion. Fortunately, a move to a reintegration of the Ottawa Charter and lifestyle approaches has begun with a a people centred approach to health promotion which focuses on personal and community development[17,18]. More generally, this approach seeks to build ecologically and economically self-reliant local economies interlinked as part of a global system.

10.3.3 Ecological public health

The term 'ecological public health' emerged from a perception of the need to integrate health and the environment[19,20]. The survival of humanity depends on the development of an ecological balance between humans and the biosphere. Globally this balance requires a rate of resource and energy use at a level of about one-fifth of that of modern high technology societies, raising fundamental questions about the type of society required for the future[21]. As with the term 'new public health', there is little need for the term 'ecological public health' as public health is, by definition, ecological. 'Public health' is an evolving term; the addition of new labels is sometimes confusing and often unnecessary. Ideally, public health should be dynamic and flexible, incorporating the most appropriate elements of earlier public health movements: disease prevention, health promotion, health education, health policy, environmental concern and community empowerment.

10.4 A critical connection: public health and epidemiology

At its formal beginnings in the middle of the nineteenth century, epidemiology was intimately linked with the public health movement. Indeed, improvement in the public's health was the justification for the foundation of the London Epidemiological Society in 1850. As we have seen, however, epidemiology has become divorced from public health practice and policy[22].

For epidemiology to become reintegrated with public health practice, changes will be required in both the education and training of epidemiologists, and in the practice of public health. These issues are addressed in the 'Leeds Declaration' which contains ten principles for action on public health research and practice[3]. This declaration supports the development of new theory and practice in epidemiology, but also acknowledges the contribution of social sciences and other disciplines to public health and the importance of the lay perspective[23]. It will not be easy for epidemiology to regain its whole population purpose and closer connection with healthy public policy; 'a social policy approach to healthy lifestyles' rather than the current 'lifestyle approach to social policy' is required[24].

There is now sufficient evidence to support the population approach to prevention. Risk factors are normally distributed and the majority of new events occur in people in the middle range of the distribution; the small proportion of the population at high risk of disease produces only a minority of the new cases of disease. A major difficulty, however, with the population wide strategy, is the prevention paradox: 'a preventive measure that brings large benefits to the community affords little to each participating individual'[25]. The high risk strategy is attractive because it yields a large benefit to sick or high risk individuals, although it affords little benefit to the community as a whole and does little to prevent epidemics. A difficult task for epidemiologists is to focus attention on strategies for whole populations and this requires advocacy.

There is potential for making strategies directed at individuals more effective with the increasing recognition that clinical decisions should be based on
measures of absolute risk rather than relative risk, that is, the actual risk of
disease an individual faces should be an important consideration in the
patient's decision about therapeutic options. With the development of clinical guidelines based on sound epidemiological data, epidemiology is changing clinical practice. For example modern guidelines for the treatment of
mild hypertension encourage the treatment of older people, especially those
with other risk factors, rather than middle-aged people[26].

Epidemiology, along with the other disciplines of public health, is indispensable to the process of health policy formation. A closer integration of
public health sciences with policy making will ensure that health policy is
influenced by evidence, just as clinical medicine is moving towards an evidence based approach[27]. If new policies are accompanied by a statement of
the supporting evidence, the policy process will become more transparent.

10.5 A growing foundation: public health education and training

Although postgraduate public health education has a long history in the
United States of America and the United Kingdom, dating back to early
this century, in most of the world public health education is a relatively new
development and funding for public health training is limited. The separation of public health from medical schools had a deleterious impact on both
schools of public health and medical schools[28]. The former became
divorced from medicine and the latter could safely neglect public health. On
both accounts, the health of the public suffered.

Public health education is developing in many countries and new schools
and institutes of public health have been established[29]. In Australia the
resurgence began in the mid-1980s stimulated by the election of a Labour
government and a review of public health education[30]. In Germany and
Eastern Europe developments occurred in the early 1990s[30,31]; prior to these
developments, Germany had no experience with postgraduate studies in
public health.

There were 54 schools of public health in Europe by 1992 most of which
were stand-alone research and training institutions or departments of
public health within a medical school[32]. Innovative broad based institutional initiatives which are closely related to public health practice are
rare[33]. There are now 27 schools of public health in the United States of
America (and 126 medical schools), five of which have been established in
the last decade. Many are developing innovative links with local depart-

ments of public health and with community organisations. The enormous growth in research grants, however, has overshadowed commitment to teaching and community practice.

Where strong schools of public health exist, closer ties with medical schools and local departments of public health are desirable. This integration is especially important in poor countries which cannot afford either an elite medical profession modelled on European or North American lines, or a weak public health profession. The hope that the public health approach would permeate medical schools has, so far, proved illusory. Changing the dominant philosophy of medical schools will be difficult, especially if they remain isolated from their communities; few medical schools have responsibility for the health and health care needs of their local communities. On the other hand, if medical schools embrace public health and establish close links with their communities, public health will flourish. Of central importance is that public health sees itself as a specialty in its own right and not as a speciality of medicine.

The development of public health training accreditation systems to ensure public accountability for the training activities is a priority in all countries. Such systems can be developed collegially and constructively using peer review[34].

In the short term, it matters little where public health professionals are trained; the nature of their training and their orientation are paramount. A key goal is the strengthening of the partnership between the two processes of education and practice[35]. The appropriate institutional base will be determined by local and national history and current practicalities. Whatever the base, strong institutional support and leadership of public health education and training is essential to bridge the gulf between academic and practical public health and to ensure that students are socialised in the values of public health.

10.6 The promise of public health research

Public health research has been one important contributor to the increase in life expectancy over the last century. There is still much more to be learnt, however, and much knowledge awaits implementation. Public health research is a multi-disciplinary activity. It involves the application of the whole range of biological, social and behavioural sciences to the health problems of human populations. All too often, however, it is limited to epidemiological and health systems research. The real research challenge is the exploration of the interaction between social factors and disease.

Public health research is underfunded and researchers are in short supply[36]. Globally, about US$55 billion is spent on health research overall, with only about 10% spent on researching the health needs of poor countries[37]. In Australia less than 2% of total health expenditure was spent on health research and development in 1990–91 and less than a quarter of this went on public health research[38]. In New Zealand the proportion of health related research expenditure directed to public health is similar; the relative underspending on public health research was one justification for transforming the Medical Research Council into the Health Research Council of New Zealand. This transformation had a beneficial impact on public health research funding. Innovative methods of funding public health research are required in order to rapidly build effective multi-disciplinary research groups.

At the international level, the World Bank and WHO have identified research topics which have the potential to contribute rapidly to health improvements. The major public health research challenges identified include:

- the continuing epidemics of preventable childhood infectious diseases which are aggravated by poverty and undernutrition;
- the economic, social and environmental changes which lead to emerging and re-emerging infectious diseases;
- the growing epidemics of non-communicable diseases and injuries; and
- the assessment of the effectiveness and efficiency of public health programmes.

This exercise, which built upon the 1993 World Bank Report *Investing in Health*[39], will shape the long-term priorities of the main international health research agencies. Regrettably, the emphasis is on disease-specific interventions and 'best buy' packages at the expense of broad social and public health programmes which deal with the underlying causes of premature death and disease[37].

Much public health and epidemiological research has become repetitive and divorced from both practice and problem solving. Closer integration of public health agencies and academic institutions will improve the quality and relevance of public health research. Public health researchers will increase their relevance to the needs of policy makers if they pay more attention to the policy environment and the process of policy making[40]. Some of the irrelevance of public health research would be overcome if research adhered to the motto of an independent research organisation, the

New England Research Institutes, which reads 'no research without thera-peutic or policy benefit'[41].

The value of using the appropriate research method for the appropriate question is now recognised[42,43]. As epidemiology moves from a focus on individual risk factors and towards the more difficult task of exploring community influences and social and economic structures, it will need to work much more closely with other public health sciences. The great strength of qualitative research is that it has the potential to illuminate the nature of quantitative relationships. Similarly, medical and biological sci-entists are essential for good public health research[44].

10.7 Public health advocacy: an important skill

A key aspect of public health practice is advocacy[45]. All countries require a strong advocacy group for public health, yet few have an established and vigorous public health association that takes advocacy seriously. The American Public Health Association, the Canadian Public Health Association, and the Australian Public Health Association are examples of agencies that have good visibility and an impact on health policy. Regional groups such as the recently proposed Union for Hanseatic Public Health[46] are also useful.

Public health scientists, in comparison with their medical colleagues, have a low public profile; public health is not a public relations success. Too often, public health practitioners are portrayed as moralists preaching against pleasurable behaviours such as drinking and smoking. In addition, public health practitioners, unskilled in media advocacy, are reticent to take credit for their contributions to health improvements. Extravagant claims and promises from laboratory sciences and clinical medicine are often left unchallenged and journalists occasionally let their enthusiasm overshadow balanced reporting[47].

Public health practitioners must work constructively with the media which have an impressive influence on policy debates[48,49]. The strategic use of mass media to advance a social or policy initiative is a powerful public health tool and can be used to strengthen community action. Media advo-cacy functions by setting agendas, framing debates, and stressing the need for policy solutions to personal problems. Tobacco control activists have, on occasions, been particularly successful as media advocates[50].

Advocacy is especially difficult for public health practitioners employed by government agencies. Practitioners employed by more independent agencies such as universities have a special responsibility to speak publicly on the underlying causes of population health levels and the most appropriate public health strategies. One solution is for government employed public health practitioners to form advocacy groups which act outside the confines of the bureaucracy.

10.8 Participation: the key to a strong public health movement

Public participation is the key to a strong and vigorous public health movement. True participation implies effective two-way consultation and joint ownership of public health programmes[51]. Much of this work is unrecognised, at least in economic terms, as it is unpaid and undertaken largely by women. Public health practitioners need to appreciate the existence of popular beliefs about disease causation and occurrence. For example, members of the public put a greater emphasis on the role of 'stress' and often invoke fatalism to explain death and disease[52]. A top-down approach to health promotion is unlikely to be effective as it ignores the active way in which people construct explanations of health and disease[53].

The Alma Ata declaration recognised that 'people have the right to participate individually and collectively in the planning and implementation of their health care'[12]. A major challenge is to encourage effective participation in countries in which involvement in public affairs is rare. The poor remain poor because they are marginalised from the political and economic decision making process. Poor people take no part in the allocation of health resources or in the more general allocation of public resources. Economic and social decisions are inevitably, but unfairly, more influenced by powerful and entrenched vested interest.

Global progress in public health is closely related to the development of mass participatory democracy beginning at the community level and extending throughout society. The basis of social cohesiveness and democracy are co-operative civic networks[54]. The experience of the few countries which have achieved high population levels of health at relatively low cost, emphasises the need for a strong social consensus on the importance of health and educational services. This in turn often reflects a vigorous democracy, especially at the local level[55]. Unfortunately, the prospects for democratic participation in much of the world is bleak. Public health practitioners must continue to stress the need for this participation and to advocate with the communities they serve[56].

Public health practioners must also take a leadership role in keeping the public health vision alive, rather than awaiting the spontaneous development of mass movements for public health. In many countries environmental issues are the impetus for building a public health constituency. Public health researchers and practitioners can foster the development of a community voice by forming close links with community groups. This is easier when the research stems directly from community concerns. There is often a fine line between community participation and community manipulation. Inevitably, health promotion challenges established power bases; enduring successes will only occur when there is a strong alignment between community concerns and public health policy.

10.9 Public health, human rights and ecological constraints

Although the modern origins of the idea of human rights go back at least as far as the eighteenth century, health as a human right is a relatively recent concept[57]. The United Nations in 1948 adopted the Universal Declaration of Human Rights which includes a statement that 'everyone has the right to a standard of living adequate for the health and well being of himself and his family'. This right was further expanded by the United Nations in 1966 in an International Covenant on Economic, Social and Cultural Rights (Article 12) which included the obligation for states ratifying the covenant to take steps to:

* reduce stillborn and infant mortality rates;
* promote the healthy development of the child;
* improve all aspects of environmental and industrial hygiene; and
* prevent, treat, and control epidemic, endemic, occupational and other diseases.

These general statements, although important and legally binding in international law, do not make it easy to determine the specific obligations involved[58]. Signatories are obliged to work towards achieving these rights, by adopting legislative measures, but progress is limited because action is conditional on the availability of resources (Article 2).

The formation of the World Health Organization provided the first international agency to lead the movement for health as a human right. WHO's constitution proclaims 'the enjoyment of the highest attainable standard of health is one of the fundamental rights of every human being' and WHO's objective is 'the attainment by all peoples of the highest possible level of health'. The legal implications of the WHO definition of health are that nations have duties both to promote health, social and related services as well as to prevent or remove barriers to the realisation and maintenance of health[59].

International and national statements on health as a human right mean little when there is no enforceable mechanism for making them effective. Even where legal mechanisms are available, they are not often used. These statements, however, have tremendous symbolic value. Unfortunately, fewer than 30 countries have an agency responsible for human rights and very few of these agencies have any responsibility for health. Furthermore, most international statements have a strong 'western' flavour and assume the equality of men and women; many religious and cultural groups do not acknowledge this equality. While equity in opportunities for health is an important public health goal, it is obvious that this view is not widely held in most countries. Public health professionals are able to point out the consequences of ignoring equity in health as a fundamental human goal.

10.9.1 Principles of public health ethics

The four basic principles of medical care ethics also apply to the practice of public health: respect for autonomy, non-maleficence, beneficence, and justice, as described in Chapter 6. From a public health perspective, all four principles are important, but public health practice is fundamentally different from medical practice. In general people seek advice and help from doctors and other health care professionals; few ask for public health advice. In the interests of beneficence, the principle of 'doing the most good', public health practitioners make judgements about healthy lifestyles and thus run the risk of paternalism. Public health practitioners, and especially health promotors, will achieve more by focusing on the provision of health enabling conditions and opportunities.

Issues of rights are involved in all aspects of public health programmes from analysis to implementation and monitoring. Each stage can involve a conflict of rights, for example, rights to privacy versus access to data for epidemiological purposes. The moral basis for public health interventions is not always explicit and ranges from a desire to inform people by health education, to the promotion of the 'common good' through policy advocacy[60]. There is always tension in public health between autonomy of the individual and the desire to protect and promote the health of the whole population. All public health programmes attempt to balance individual and collective rights.

Public health and human rights are linked in three general ways[61]. Firstly, public health policies can have both a positive and negative impact on human rights, especially when state power is used to limit the 'rights of a few for the good of many', as is often the case in the control of communicable disease; however, there need not be a conflict between human rights and public health. For example, the control of the HIV/AIDS pandemic requires increased attention to the promotion of the human rights of people most at risk of infection. AIDS is inextricable from individual and collective behaviour, strongly influenced by broad social forces, and directly linked with social discrimination. Little progress will be made in reducing the risk of HIV transmission until discrimination on the basis of sexual preference is legally prohibited and antidiscrimination measures and educational programmes are widely promoted and enforced.

The second link is the health impact of violations of human rights. Unfortunately, there is all too much evidence to support this linkage, ranging from medically sanctioned and culturally accepted torture, genital mutilation of girls, or the systematic rape and elimination of refugees or political opponents.

The third, and most fundamental consideration, is that health and human rights are inextricably linked in the struggle to advance human well-being within the context of the closed biosphere[62]. To die because of the absence of the fundamentals of health, whether it be medical care or adequate nutrition, is a violation of human rights. The striking and enduring inequalities in health within, and especially between, countries is both a public health and a human rights issue. The reduction of inequalities represents a great opportunity for improving the health of all populations, but this goal will require both public health and social policy interventions. Public health practitioners have a responsibility to draw attention to the importance of the linkage between human rights and public health and to develop methods of assessing the impact on human rights of health policies and programmes and health reforms[63].

10.10 The internationalisation of public health

10.10.1 The daunting global context

A major challenge facing public health is to sustain and extend the health gains that have been made over the last half century, a daunting task. Several interrelated global developments have a profound influence on public health:

- the exploitative relationship between wealthy and poor countries;
- the prevailing ideology which stresses the role of the 'free market' and 'individualism'; and
- the threats to the environment.

The globalisation of the economy, with attendant changes in world trade and the spread of free market policies and service based economies, will be completed by the end of the century. The security of the globalised economy is far from guaranteed, as evidenced by the recent economic problems in Mexico and other South American countries, and the ongoing problem in much of sub-Saharan Africa. The marked inequality in wealth between countries is firmly rooted in the exploitative relationship between rich and poor countries, with poor countries viewed largely as a market for the products of wealthy countries and as a source of cheap labour. Indeed, the rich countries have achieved their wealth by exploiting the poverty of the poor[64]. The extent of global poverty, poor nutrition, the debt crisis, and the deterioration of the environment all demand attention, as does population growth which interacts with poverty to aggravate the environmental pressures.

In the face of these problems, current development aid for poor countries is both grossly inadequate and irrelevant, especially when it is tied to conformity to free trade, economic growth and individual liberty. Wealthy countries have repeatedly pledged to give at least 0.7% of GNP to official development assistance programmes, yet only a few countries, Norway, Sweden, Denmark and the Netherlands, have achieved this modest goal[65].

The health impact of the new World Trade Organisation initiated in 1994 by 118 countries is yet to be determined. The prospects are not promising. It is likely that poor people will be further exposed to the effects of the global marketplace in return for their cheap labour. Global forces can also severely limit the public health policy options at a national level. For example, the health policies of many countries are constrained by the conditions imposed by the World Bank and the International Monetary Fund; the World Bank is now, in financial terms, the most important agency in world health[66]. The international governmental agencies (such as the World Health Organization) and non-governmental organizations are relatively powerless by comparison.

Since 1945 at least five United Nations organisations have become heavily involved in international health activities: WHO, World Bank, UN Children's Fund (UNICEF), UN Population Fund (UNFPA), and UN Development Programme (UNDP). Although WHO still regards itself as the lead agency, this view is not shared by other agencies and there is serious lack of co-ordination and co-operation among agencies[67].

The World Bank puts much faith in the involvement of the private sector in the provision of health care in poor countries. The route to good health, as envisaged by the World Bank, is through economic development and medical science. In this sense, the World Bank is increasingly influencing international health. Although the World Bank's 1993 report *Investing in Health* recognises that poverty and ill health are causally related, it does not advocate the redistribution of wealth as a means of improving health[68]. The WHO Health For All emphasis on a broad social and economic approach is not endorsed by the World Bank; nor is the importance of debt relief for poor countries explicitly addressed. The 1995 World Development Report, however, does mark a shift away from the World Bank's long-term *laissez-faire* doctrine. The Bank now acknowledges that massive inequalities are a barrier to rising prosperity and growth and recognises the need for strong trade unions and greater equality in poor countries[69].

The World Bank also advocates the use of specific cost effective interventions. This approach is reminiscent of 'magic bullet' medicine which attempted to identify pharmaceutical agents for each disease. The strongest contender for the 'public health magic bullet' is the education of women. While the World Bank deserves credit for stressing the importance of education, the social and cultural barriers which limit the opportunities for girls and young women also need to be addressed.

10.10.2 WHO: in need of reform

Health problems have never respected national boundaries and most health issues need co-ordinated international action. There is a desperate need for strong global leadership for health. WHO for several decades after its founding in 1948, provided this leadership. During its first three decades, WHO focused successfully on providing scientific and technical advice and setting international standards. It reached its highest standing with the smallpox eradication campaign, successfully completed in 1977 and formally certified in 1979. Partial victory at minimal cost has also been achieved in WHO's campaign to eradicate guineaworm disease by 1995[70]. The success to date towards the eradication of polio is also a great credit to WHO, although momentum may be slipping as the target date (the year 2000) approaches[71,72]; in at least 15 countries polio eradication will be especially difficult because the health infrastructure has been severely weakened by armed conflict and civil strife.

In the early 1980s, WHO provided a second round of leadership by firmly advocating a broad vision of health under the banner of Health For All by the Year 2000; this advocacy led the Organization into politically sensitive areas. A fundamental weakness of efforts to implement the Health For All philosophy is the assumption that equity in health can be achieved by health services and narrowly defined disease prevention and health promotion activities. Although the Health for All vision and rhetoric were initially broad and encompassed social and economic change, selective primary care rapidly became the prime strategy followed by a rapid retreat from the comprehensive Health for All strategies. Abundant evidence demonstrates that this approach will not achieve equity[57]. Unfortunately, the unattainability of the Health For All goal may indirectly have weakened the Organization. The rhetoric has not been matched by the achievements of the Organization, only in part because of insufficient resources[73]. Over the last decade the vision has faded and the status of WHO has declined.

The serious criticisms levelled at WHO, both centrally and regionally, indicate that the Organization is at a critical point: either it reforms or it becomes increasingly irrelevant. Lack of effective leadership, confused vision, poor accountability, and an unwieldy bureaucratic structure have all contributed to the Organization's inability to translate policy into action[73]. The Regional Office for Africa in particular has received strong criticism from WHO's external auditor for deficiencies in accounting methods and weak management controls[74]. The power of member states to promote vested interests and to lobby for political appointments has led to fragmented programmes and a poorly defined set of priorities. WHO's country operations are limited because it must work through national health ministries. Furthermore, WHO has little money to spend at the country level and much of its impact is indirect and takes years to be apparent. In 1993 WHO declared tuberculosis to be a 'global health emergency'; although this was the first time WHO had singled out any disease in such a manner, it has not allocated resources commensurate with the emergency[75].

Undoubtedly, many areas of high achievement continue in WHO, especially in the special programmes supported by extra budgetary funds from the wealthiest member states[76]. These funds provide a way for donors to support programmes outside the management's control. Unfortunately, this has led to competition for both funding and implementation at the country level which in turn has undermined the process of developing integrated primary health care systems in many poor countries[77]. Some of the extra budgetary donors are no longer continuing their high level of support because of dissatisfaction with the lack of reforms in the Organization. For example, in 1995 Sweden, the second largest contributor of extra budgetary funds after the United States of America, reduced its extra budgetary support by half and in future years will reduce it even further if major reforms are not implemented[78]. Denmark's Parliament recently halved the country's contribution to WHO as a gesture of dissatisfaction with the top leadership[79].

Training health professionals is one of WHO's major strategies for improving health care in the poor world, yet even this programme lacks a strategy and structure and is seen by some as a route for channelling donated money back to wealthy countries[80]. Research capacity building, another WHO initiative, is itself an under-developed and under-researched activity[81]. Institutions in wealthy countries will continue to play an important part in training and conducting research with students and professionals from poor countries; but other models exist. For example, the International Clinical Epidemiology Network (INCLEN) which concentrates on building a critical mass of multi-disciplinary researchers in poor countries provides ongoing support, both scientific and financial[28].

It is imperative that WHO returns to articulating a realistic and shared vision of public health which includes a comprehensive primary health care system and an integrated intersectoral approach to health. Whilst awaiting this new vision[82], the process of revitalising WHO should continue[83]. The 1995 World Health Report, with its focus on the devastating health effects of poverty, suggests that WHO may be rediscovering its powerful advocacy voice for a broad view of health. The WHO's Ninth General Programme of Work for the period 1996–2001 is based on the Health For All model[84], another positive sign. It is unlikely that confidence will be reaffirmed in WHO until a new Organizational structure is in place and the perceived lack of leadership resolved[73,83]. The governance of WHO will also require modification to ensure that national and regional political issues no longer distort the priorities of the organisation. The role of WHO would be clarified by a joint review of the mandates of all UN agencies involved in international health programmes[67]. A reorganised and refocused WHO under new leadership will, hopefully, attract the necessary international support and funds and alleviate the chronic uncertainty in funding which had defeated past efforts at planning and management[85]. Major new initiatives are required to restore confidence in WHO.

10.11 Prospects for public health: cautious optimism

There is good reason to be cautiously optimistic about the future prospects for public health. Major improvements have taken place in global standards of health in the last half century. Health conditions have improved more in the past 50 years than in the whole of previous human history. Life expectancy has increased in almost all countries and most of the improvement in population health status in poor countries has been a result of government leadership and social and public health interventions.

On a less positive note, the twentieth century is ending in confusing global disorder[64]. The 'new world order' of the 1990s is, in general, not conducive to public health. The global economy is increasingly integrated under the banner of 'free trade' and 'market forces'. The crisis over the safety of British beef and the potential threat to public health from the link between bovine spongiform encephalopathy and Creutzfeldt–Jakob disease is a specific example of the unintended adverse effects of neo-liberal economic theory. At least some of the responsibility for the crisis can be traced to the government policy of deregulation which allowed cattle to be fed meat rendered from sheep infected with scrapie[86].

Although overall levels of health are improving, there are still marked variations in health between and within regions, and social class variations in health are increasing in many countries. The poorest 50 nations are home to a fifth of the world's population, but have seen their share of world income drop to 2%[87]. Even in the United States of America, one-seventh of the population in 1992 was poor[88]. The situation in Central and Eastern European countries is particularly bleak[89].

Global challenges to health, apart from market forces, are mounting. The dominance of the ideology of individualism causes serious difficulties for the collective actions which are the core of effective public health policy and programmes. The response to widespread environmental damage has so far been minimal. Our vulnerability to disease could readily be exposed by subtle environmental changes or a breakdown in basic public health services. New diseases, such as AIDS, expose the sharp divisions within society and the abuse of human rights. The control of 'old' diseases such as tuberculosis is limited by drug resistance, limited funding, inadequate strategies and lack of attention to the underlying social conditions[90].

The global burden of non-communicable diseases will inevitably increase as populations age. Population growth remains excessive in many parts of the world and reinforces poverty. The threat posed by the ongoing spread of nuclear weapons is precariously controlled and the dissemination of small scale weapons of destruction is out of control[91,92]. Civil wars continue unabated, aggravated by ethnic and religious rivalries, especially in Africa but also in Central and Eastern Europe and the Middle East. In short, the struggle to improve the health of the public will be never ending as new threats and problems emerge.

In the absence of a strong and cohesive international movement, public health is ill-equipped to face these challenges. Public health education and research are poorly organised and inadequately funded at both national and international levels; undergraduate and non-tertiary public health education are poorly developed. The public health work force is fragmented. Internationally, public health under the influence of the World Bank is increasingly defined as selected technical interventions against a limited range of diseases.

Public health competes with other values, such as liberty and material prosperity. Fortunately, health is compatible with other important and inclusive social goals, especially conserving the environment. The realisation that a high degree of wealth is not essential for a healthy population leads to the challenges of ensuring 'health at low cost' and a more equitable distribution of the available wealth. A priority for public health practitioners is to have health as a social goal, high on the political agenda, at the same time avoiding prescribing 'healthy lifestyles'. People will then make choices, especially around issues of consumption, fully informed of the health consequences for them as individuals and for society as a whole.

Opportunities exist for the public health movement to exert a more central role in human affairs. The economic pendulum will swing back towards a more collectivist approach as the ill-effects of the free market are recognised, especially by the huge marginalised segments of the world's population. Public health practitioners, however, cannot passively await a more favourable political environment.

In many countries postgraduate education in public health is undergoing a renaissance and new leadership will emerge from the ranks of these students. Public health service agencies increasingly welcome newly trained graduates in public health. Participatory public health research is also increasing, especially around local environmental issues and among indigenous people. The major public health research issues concerning the impact of global environmental change are under active investigation by multidisciplinary teams. The need for integration of research methods is widely recognised and linkages are being developed between public health education and research institutions and policy agencies.

A heavy responsibility rests on current public health practitioners. If, at this critical stage in the evolution of public health, we choose the narrow, individualistic path of least resistance, we will become marginalised as, at best, a poor relation of clinical medicine. If, on the other hand, we choose a broad and inclusive vision of public health and translate this into practice, there is a real prospect for a true 'golden age of public health'. Above all is the need for a collective, international responsibility that addresses the requirements of future generations through co-ordinated multi-sectoral action at local, community, national, regional and international levels. If public health practitioners are successful in framing these debates and communicating their importance, public support for public health activities will increase and reduce the threats to public health.

10.12 Conclusion

For global public health movements to claim a central position in public policy, several actions must be taken. An international debate is required to reach a consensus on the broad scope of public health, its theoretical underpinning and its ethical and moral basis. Epidemiology and the other public health sciences must reclaim their close linkages with public health policy and practice. Public health professionals must recognise that evidence based advocacy is a legitimate public health activity which must be taught and practised by all public health professionals. A strong public health movement will require community participation in setting the public health research agenda. Above all, given the interdependence of global political and socioeconomic movements, strong international leadership is required.

Chapter 10   Key Points

- The global context for public health is daunting.
- Strong international leadership is required because of the global nature of the threats to public health.
- Public health is at the crossroads: the choice is between a narrow focus on individual health issues or a broad focus on the major health determinants and problems.
- If public health practitioners adopt a broad focus and implement appropriate strategies, there are good prospects for a true 'golden age of public health'.

References

1. Winslow CEA. Public health at the crossroads. *Am J Pub Hlth* 1926; **16**:1075–85.
2. Beaglehole R, Davis P. Setting national health goals and targets in the context of a fiscal crisis: the politics of social choice in New Zealand. *Int J Hlth Serv* 1992; **22**:417–28.
3. Anon. Population health looking upstream. *Lancet* 1994; **343**:429–30.
4. Graham H. Women's smoking and family health. *Soc Sci Med* 1987; **25**:47–56.
5. Nijhuis HGJ, Van Der Maesen LJG. The philosophical foundations of

public health: an invitation to debate. *J Epidemiol Comm Hlth* 1994; **48**:1–3.

6. Seedhouse D. The way around health economics' dead end. *Hlth Care Anal* 1995; **3**:205–20.

7. Hill HW. *The New Public Health*. New York: Macmillan, 1916.

8. Ashton J, Seymour H. *The New Public Health*. Milton Keynes: Open University Press, 1988.

9. Lalonde M. *A New Perspective on the Health of Canadians*. Ottawa: National Health and Welfare, 1974.

10. US Department of Health Education and Welfare. *Healthy People. The Surgeon General's Report on Health Promotion and Disease Prevention.* DHEW Pub No 79–55071. Washington: US Public Health Service, 1979.

11. McGinnis JM. Setting objectives for public health in the 1990s: experience and prospects. *Ann Rev Publ Hlth* 1990; 11:231–49.

12. World Health Organization. *Alma-Ata. Primary Health Care (Health For All Series No.1)*. Geneva: World Health Organization, 1978.

13. Walsh JA, Warren KS. Selective primary health care: an interim strategy for disease control in developing countries. *New Engl J Med* 1979; **301**:967–74.

14. Rifkin SB, Walt G. Why health improves: defining the issues concerning 'comprehensive primary health care' and 'selective primary health care'. *Soc Sci Med* 1986; **6**:559–66.

15. Ottawa Charter for Health Promotion. *Hlth Prom* 1992; **1**:i-v.

16. Baum FE. Healthy cities and change: social movement or bureaucratic tool? *Hlth Prom Int* 1993; **8**:31–40.

17. Dougherty CJ. Bad faith and victim-blaming: the limits of health promotion. *Hlth Care Anal* 1993; **1**:111–19.

18. Raeburn J, Rootman I. *People-Centred Health Promotion*. London: John Wiley, 1997.

19. World Commission on Environment and Development. *Our Common Future*. Oxford: Oxford University Press, 1987.

20. World Health Organization Commission on Health and the Environment. *Our Planet, Our Health*. Geneva: WHO, 1992.

21. Boyden S, Shirlow M. Ecological sustainability and the quality of life. In: Brown V (ed.). *2020: A Sustainable Healthy Future. Towards an Ecology of Health*. Melbourne: La Trobe University, 1989.

22. Pearce N. Traditional epidemiology, modern epidemiology, and public health. *Am J Pub Hlth* 1996; **86**:678–83.

23. Davison C, Smith GD, Frankel S. Lay epidemiology and the prevention paradox: the implications of coronary candidacy for health education. *Soc Hlth Illn* 1991; **13**:1–19.

24. McKinlay JB. Paradigmatic obstacles to improvements in women's health. *Paper presented at the Symposium on Women's Health*, Puerto Rico, USA. December 1994.

25. Rose G. *The Strategy of Preventive Medicine*. Oxford: Oxford University Press, 1992.

26. Jackson R, Barham P, Bills J, Birch T, McLennan D, MacMahon S, Maling T. The management of raised blood pressure in New Zealand. *Br Med J* 1993; **307**:107–10

27. Ham C, Hunter DJ, Robinson R. Evidence based policymaking: research must inform health policy as well as medical care. *Br Med J* 1995; **310**:71–2.

28. White KL. *Healing the Schism. Epidemiology, Medicine, and the Public's Health*. New York: Springer, 1991.

29. Ashton J. Institutes of public health and medical schools: grasping defeat from the jaws of victory? *J Epidemiol Comm Hlth* 1992; **46**:165–8.
30. Jamrozik K. A glimpse at public health in Eastern Europe. *Aust J Publ Hlth* 1994; **19**:102–3.
31. Kolip P, Schott T. The postgraduate public health training programs in Germany. In: Laaser U, de Leeuw E, Stock C (eds). *Scientific Foundations for a Public Health Policy in Europe*. Weinheim: Juventa, 1996.
32. De Leeuw E. European schools of public health in state of flux. *Lancet* 1995; **345**:1158–60.
33. Navarro V. European schools of public health. *Lancet* 1995; **345**:1511.
34. Public Health Accreditation project. *The Final Report of the Accreditation Working Party*. Canberra: Commonwealth Department of Human Services and Health, 1995.
35. Rotem A, Walters J, Dewdney J. The public health workforce education and training study. *Aust J Pub Hlth* 1995; **19**:437–8.
36. Holland WW, Fitzsimons B, O'Brien M. 'Back to the future' – public health research into the next century. *J Pub Hlth Med* 1994; **16**:4–10.
37. World Health Organization Ad Hoc Committee on Health Research Relating to Future Intervention Options. *Investing in Health Research and Development*. Geneva: WHO, 1995.
38. Nichol W, McNeice K, Goss J (eds). *Expenditure on health research and development in Australia. Welfare Division Working Paper No. 7*. Canberra: Australian Institute Health & Welfare, 1994.
39. World Development Report. *Investing in Health, World Development Indicators*. New York: Oxford University Press, 1993.
40. Walt G. How far does research influence policy? *Eur J Pub Hlth* 1994; **4**:233–5.
41. Network: The newsletter of the New England Research Institutes. Summer/Fall 1995.
42. Black N. Why we need qualitative research. *J Epidemiol Comm Hlth* 1994; **48**: 425–6.
43. Baum F. Researching public health: behind the qualitative-quantitative methodological debate. *Soc Sci Med* 1995; **40**:459–68.
44. Holland WW. The hazards of epidemiology. *Am J Pub Hlth* 1995; **85**:616–7.
45. Weed DL. Science, ethics guidelines, and advocacy in epidemiology. *Ann Epidemiol* 1994; **4**:166–71.
46. Vuori H. A new Hanseatic Union for public health? *Eur J Pub Hlth* 1994; **4**:153–5.
47. Anon. SIDS theory: from hype to reality. *Lancet* 1995; **346**:1503.
48. Wallack L. Media advocacy: a strategy for empowering people and communties. *J Pub Hlth Pol* 1994; **15**:420–35.
49. Chapman S, Lupton D. *The Fight For Public Health: Principles and Practice of Media Advocacy*. London: Br Med J Publishing Group, 1994.
50. Chapman S. A David and Goliath Story: tobacco advertising in Australia. *Br Med J* 1980; **281**:1187–90.
51. Scally G. Citizen health. *Lancet* 1996; **347**:3–4
52. Davison C, Frankel S, Smith GD. The limits of lifestyle: re-assessing fatalism in the popular culture of illness prevention. *Soc Soc Med* 1992; **34**:675–85.
53. Bury M. Health promotion and lay epidemiology: a sociological view. *Hlth Care Analysis* 1994; **2**:23–30.

54. Putnam RD, Leonardi R, Nanetti RY. *Making Democracy Work*. Princeton: Princeton University Press, 1993.
55. Caldwell JC. Routes to low mortality in poor countries. *Pop Dev Review* 1986; **12**:171–220.
56. Labonte R. A holosphere of healthy and sustainable communities. *Aust J Pub Hlth* 1993; **17**:4–12.
57. Susser M. Health as a human right: an epidemiologist's perspective on the public health. *Am J Pub Hlth* 1993; **83**:418–26.
58. Leary V. The right to health in international human rights law. *Human Rights* 1994; **1**:24–57.
59. Cook RJ. *Women's Health and Human Rights. The Promotion and Protection of Women's Health through International Human Rights Law*. Geneva: World Health Organization, 1994.
60. Cole P. The moral bases for public health interventions. *Epidemiology* 1994; **6**:78–83.
61. Mann J, Gostin L, Gruskin S, Brennan T, Lazzarini Z, Fineberg HV. Health and human rights. *Hlth Human Rights* 1994; **1**:6–23.
62. McMichael AJ. Contemplating a one child world. *Br Med J* 1995; **311**:1651–2.
63. Gostin L, Mann J. Towards the development of a human rights impact assessment for the formulation and evaluation of health policies. *Hlth Human Rights* 1994; **1**:58–81.
64. Hobsbawm E. *Age of Extremes: The Short Twentieth Century, 1914–1991*. London: Michael Joseph, 1994.
65. UNICEF. *The State of the World's Children*. New York: Oxford University Press, 1995.
66. Editorial. The World Bank, listening and learning. *Lancet* 1996; **347**:411
67. Lee K, Collinson S, Walt G, Gilson L. Who should be doing what in international health: a confusion of mandates in the United Nations? *Br Med J* 1996; **312**:302–7
68. O'Keefe E. The World Bank: health policy, poverty and equity. *Crit Public Hlth* 1995; **6**:3:28–35.
69. Elliott L. World Bank to ease *laissez-faire* policy. *The Guardian Weekly*, April 9, 1992:12.
70. Caincross S. Victory over guineaworm disease: partial or pyrrhic? *Lancet* 1995; **346**:1440.
71. Hull HF, Ward NA, Hull BP, Milstien JB, de Quadros C. Paralytic poliomyelitis: seasoned strategies, disappearing disease. *Lancet* 1994; **343**:1331–7.
72. Hull HF, Lee JW. Sabin, Salk, or sequential? *Lancet* 1996; **347**:630.
73. Peabody JW. An organisational analysis of the World Health Organization: narrowing the gap between promise and performance. *Soc Sci Med* 1995; **40**:731–42.
74. McGregor A. Resignation of WHO external auditor. *Lancet* 1995; **345**:1228–9.
75. Reichman LB. How to ensure the continued resurgence of tuberculosis. *Lancet* 1996; **347**:175–7.
76. Vaughan JP, Mogedal S, Kruse SE, Lee K, Walt G, de Wilde K. *Cooperation For Health Development. Extra-budgetary Funds in the World Health Organization*. Australian Agency for International Development, Royal Ministy of Foreign Affairs, Norway, ODA, United Kingdom, 1995.

77. Godlee F. WHO's special programmes: undermining from above. *Br Med J* 1995; **310**:178–82.
78. McGregor A. Sweden to cut WHO funding. *Lancet* 1995; **345**:49–50.
79. Awuonda M. Danes snub WHO by reducing aid donations. *Lancet* 1995; **346**:1619.
80. Godlee F. WHO fellowships: what do they achieve? *Br Med J* 1995; **310**:110–12.
81. Trostle J. Research capacity building in international health: definitions, evaluations and strategies for success. *Soc Sci Med* 1992; **35**:1321–4.
82. Kickbusch I. World Health Organization: change and progress. *Br Med J* 1995; **310**:1518–20.
83. Smith R. The WHO: change or die. *Br Med J* 1995; **310**:543–4.
84. World Health Organization. *Ninth general programme of work covering the period 1996–2001. Health for all Series, No 9.* Geneva: WHO, 1994.
85. McGregor A. 'Chronic' cash shortage hits WHO. *Lancet* 1996; **347**:187.
86. Gray J. Nature bites back at human hubris. *Guardian Weekly*, April 7, 1996.
87. Watkins K. *The Oxfam Poverty Report.* Oxford: Oxfam, 1995.
88. Frankel DH. Measuring poverty in USA. *Lancet* 1995; **345**:1232.
89. Field MG. The health crisis in the former Soviet Union: a report from the 'post-war' zone. *Soc Sci Med* 1995; **41**:1469–78.
90. Lerner BH. New York City's tuberculosis control efforts: the historical limitations of the 'War on Consumption'. *Am J Pub Hlth* 1993; **83**:758–66.
91. Lown B. Time to leave behind genocidal weapons. *Br Med J* 1995; **310**:993–4.
92. Coupland RM. The effect of weapons on health. *Lancet* 1996; **347**:450–1.

Index